In Search of the Alzheimer's Wanderer

In Search of the Alzheimer's Wanderer

A Workbook to Protect Your Loved One

Mark L. Warner

Purdue University Press / West Lafayette, Indiana

ISBN 978-1-55753-399-9
     1-55753-399-7

CONTENTS

IN APPRECIATION

I would like to thank and acknowledge the people who were generous enough to offer their time and expertise to review *In Search of the Alzheimer's Wanderer,* including:

Mary Barnes—President and CEO of Alzheimer's Community Care, West Palm Beach, FL.

Marianne Dickerman Caldwell—Author of *Gone . . . Without a Trace*, the story of her mother, Stella Mallory Dickerman, an Alzheimer's patient who in 1991 was discovered missing.

Officer Craig B. Hall—Palm Beach County Sheriff's Department, Palm Beach, FL.

Geri Richards Hall, Ph.D., ARNP, CNS, FAAN—Advanced Practical Nurse, Director of Master's Program, Iowa College of Nursing.

Lieutenant John Kuklinski—Hollywood, Florida Fire-Rescue.

Beth Witrogen McLeod—Author of *Caregiving, The Spiritual Journey of Love, Loss and Renewal;* Pulitzer Prize nominee, former moderator of the AARP Online Caregiver Support Group, speaker and consultant on caregiving and aging issues.

Sue Matthews Petrovski—Author of *A Return Journey: Hope and Strength in the Aftermath of Alzheimer's*, a unique look at the environment of Alzheimer's—the afflicted, the affected, and the afterthoughts.

Ellen S. Warner—President of Ageless Design, Inc., Editor-in-Chief of *The Alzheimer's Daily News*, and co-founder of The Alzheimer's Store.

<u>Caregiver Advisory Committee</u>:

Adele Richards	**K. Deveau**
Pat Rummenie	**Dalton J. Nix**
Lyn Thomas	**George Stanley**

Introduction

"In Spotsylvania, VA, a 67-year-old man wandered from his home on New Year's Eve. In Oldham County, KY, a 77-year-old woman disappeared in sub-freezing temperatures in mid-January without a jacket or shoes. And yesterday, an 87-year-old resident of Watertown, CT left her home barefoot in the blizzard.

All of them suffered from Alzheimer's disease."[1]

"Most people believe that having a family member vanish will never happen to them. Those who fall victim to this trauma consequently are caught unaware about what to do. No one is exempt from the possibility of it happening to them. Each year in the United States, approximately 1.8 million persons are reported missing. Many remain missing."

—Marianne Caldwell, author of *Gone . . . Without a Trace*[2]

"If someone with dementia can walk, that person can wander and become missing.

If someone with dementia is missing, that person is lost.

If someone with dementia is lost, that person is at risk of harm."[3]

Each year there are an estimated 125,000 people with Alzheimer's disease or a related dementia who leave the safety of their home and family, unable to find their way back.[4] Most families do not believe anything so terrible, so catastrophic, could ever happen to them. They certainly do not prepare for it.

Wandering is the skeleton in the Alzheimer's closet, the lurking danger and topic that is never discussed—until it happens. Then it is too late—a family's mother, father, husband, wife, brother or sister is now missing, wandering the streets, woods, city or countryside with no idea where he or she is or how to get back. Now that person, and her life of 60, 70, 80 or 90 years, is in dire trouble. If she is not found in 24 hours, she has only about a 50-50 chance of surviving.

Yet there are steps that their families could take to help them find their loved ones, if one day or night they are discovered missing: questions whose answers could provide valuable clues to where they might go, things that attract them, immediate neighborhood dangers, and more. Answers that could save their lives.

---

1. "Alzheimer's Foundation Urges Steps to Prevent Wandering During Cold Weather," Press Release, Alzheimer's Foundation of America, January 24, 2005.
2. Marianne Dickerman Caldwell, *Gone . . . Without a Trace* (Forest Knolls, CA: Elder Books, 1995), p. 7.
3. Nina M. Silverstein, Gerald Flaherty, and Terri Salmons Tobin, *Dementia and Wandering Behavior: Concern for the Lost Elder* (New York: Springer Publishing Co., 2002).
4. R. J. Koester and D. E. Stooksbury, "Lost Alzheimer's Subjects-Profiles and Statistics," *Response* 11(4) (1992): 20–26.

Wandering is a life-threatening behavior.

It is certainly our hope that this book never becomes necessary for you. But if it does, the time that it takes to read it and answer some simple questions about your loved one could save his life.

Alzheimer's Disease

No words will ever be written that accurately describe to those of us on the outside what it is like to have a progressive neurological disease of the brain. The very best we can hope for is to learn as much as we can about this disease and strive to understand what it might be like to see through their eyes.

Alzheimer's disease progressively robs its victims of brain cells, the very tools we use to understand and process information. Imagine what it might be like to live in a world with only a partially functioning brain. It must be very confusing, frustrating and upsetting, all at the same time.

Imagine what it would be like to go for a walk or a drive and suddenly not recognize where you are or how you got there, or maybe find yourself roaming a parking lot looking for a car when you don't even recall what color it was. What could be more frightening than wandering from condominium door to door, not knowing which one is yours? With each growing moment the stress becomes greater—more information needed to be processed by an ever shrinking brain. Your only option is to continue to walk and walk—until you find something, anything, that makes sense.

These are but a few of the challenges that might confront a person with Alzheimer's disease, lost and wandering in public—in search of something he may or may not recall.

The one undeniable fact is that a person with Alzheimer's disease who is lost needs help and must be found. He cannot survive on his own and needs to be returned to the safety of his home, family and loved ones—as soon as possible.

Stages of Alzheimer's Disease

Alzheimer's is a disease of the brain. It begins with seemingly insignificant episodes of forgetfulness, eventually affecting every cognitive and bodily function, voluntary or involuntary. There are various descriptions of the stages of the disease that range from three to ten stages (including mild cognitive impairment (MCI) and end-of-life stages). It can take as little as two years to run the full course or as many as thirty years. The average is eight years.

For the purposes of simplicity and clarity, the following describes and divides Alzheimer's disease into three general stages—early, middle, and late.

The early stage of Alzheimer's disease is marked by occasional to regular episodes of forgetfulness—difficulty finding words, the inability to remember names, addresses, numbers, places and/or destinations. It may take little more than a simple, momentary distraction to lose an entire train of thought.

In the middle stage of the disease, as the brain falls further under attack, the person with AD has constant problems with anything and everything requiring thought—eating, toileting, bathing, dressing, communication, recognizing objects and people, difficulties with coordination, reacting to sudden changes, and even walking. By this stage of the journey just figuring out how to walk around an obstacle may be too great a mental task, as well as what to do when coming to the end of a street, remembering the way home or what "home" looks like, the proper clothes to put on with regard to the weather or seasonal conditions, or what to do if a speeding car is coming towards you. Wandering is now a major and life-threatening danger.

In the later stage the person progresses from having chronic difficulties with every type of activity to the brain slowing, and almost shutting down. Fewer tasks can be completed, until the brain seems to be doing almost nothing at all. People may eventually do little more than stare out into space, sit in their chair or bed, and say very little or nothing. Yet at any stage of the disease a person can get up and walk out of the door, not knowing what to do once on the other side.

Stage	Description
Early	The disease is present, yet remains in the background, not really affecting activities of daily living (ADLs)—eating, bathing, toileting, walking, and dressing—beyond periodic episodes of forgetfulness, repeated questions or stories, etc.
Middle	The disease has now progressed to where it has become a hindrance to everyday living. Struggling with the disease is now a constant battle, affecting everything from remembering how to use common objects to activities of daily living. The person repeats himself, gets lost or confused easily, and has a short attention span.
Late	In the later stages of the disease, the disease takes front stage, while the person recedes into the background. Now the disease has clearly won the battle, taking over every part of life—from talking to even recognizing the closest of friends and family. Your loved one is very confused and cannot survive without assistance.

Symptoms of the Disease

There is a saying in the field of Alzheimer's:

"When you've seen one person with Alzheimer's disease,
you've seen ONE person with Alzheimer's disease."

In other words, there are no clear rules or definitions of what a person with this disease is like or how he will behave—everyone is different.

But among the symptoms* that a person with Alzheimer's may display are:

Repeating Questions	Forgetfulness	Disorientation in Time & Place
Repeating Information	Irrational Fears	Difficulty with Multi-Sequential Tasks
Impaired Judgment	Paranoia	Inappropriate Sexual Behavior
Poor Self-Confidence	Depression	Difficulty with Walking or Balance
Lack of Cooperation	Illusions	Difficulty Finding Things
Indecisiveness	Delusions	Dressing Improperly
Personality Changes	Hallucinations	Eating Inappropriate Materials
Irrational Thought	Absentmindedness	Impaired Wayfinding
Withdrawal	Retrogenesis	Catastrophic Reactions
Disorientation	Wandering	Inability to Understand Instructions
Undressing in Public	Sundowning	Inability to Follow Directions
Agnosia	Aphasia	Apraxia

* This is not a complete list of Alzheimer's symptoms, nor do these symptoms apply to all individuals with AD.

Retrogenesis

Retrogenesis is a symptom of Alzheimer's that seems to be consistent with progression into the later stages of the disease.

The condition is described as "walking backwards in time." As the disease progresses the patient loses his short-term memory, leaving him with only his mid-term and long-term memory. In time he loses his mid-term memory, and only his long-term memory remains—leaving him living in a world based on recollections of his past. As such, the past becomes the present. (Imagine what it might be like if all of a sudden it was 1985 again, and you were 20 years younger, but everyone and everything around you remained the same.)

SHORT-TERM MEMORY   MIDTERM MEMORY   LONG-TERM MEMORY

This might explain why some people with Alzheimer's:

- Confuse a spouse for a parent or a son/daughter for one's spouse (If you are "only 40," who else could that older person with white or gray hair be?);

- Would not realize what year it is or who is president of the United States;

- Would not recognize their present home;

- Would once again speak in their primary language (if they came from another country);

- Would once again seek a childhood friend or sweetheart;
- Would again be concerned about their "children," who have long grown up;
- Might fear that people around them are enemy soldiers from a war fought years ago.

The concept of retrogenesis offers possible explanations for some of the otherwise incomprehensible behaviors seen in people in the middle and later stages of the disease. As such, some of the answers to questions in this workbook may provide family and search personnel with valuable clues and insights into your loved one's mindset and intentions—and, therefore, possible whereabouts.

Aphasia

Aphasia is the loss or reduction of the brain's ability to interpret and formulate language. Aphasia can take many forms, from minor (breaks in speech, forgetting obscure words) to severe (complete loss of language). This can dramatically impact one's ability to communicate with the wandering Alzheimer's patient. Aphasia can also result in the use of sexually explicit language, crude language, or profanity.

Given the loss of inhibition, the intense frustrations, and increasing confusion, aphasia worsens as the disease progresses, as well as under stressful situations (such as being lost, dehydrated, hungry, ill or injured).

Usually, the first evidence of language difficulty appears in naming objects, persons or tasks. A person may stall or substitute words. In the early stages, the person is aware of her worsening speech, and may develop methods of hiding the difficulty. She may ramble on or abruptly change the topic.

In moderate Alzheimer's disease, the patient begins to make mistakes, both in speaking and understanding conversation. She may not be able to appropriately answer questions, has difficulty in naming items or persons, and may answer nonsensically.

It is important to note here that persons who speak two or more languages may begin using words from their primary language when they forget the word in English (example: "pass me that, that, that naranja!"). As aphasia progresses, the speaker may use more and more of the primary language, combining a form of the two (or more) languages. Ultimately, the speaker may revert to the primary language totally, becoming completely non-responsive in English.

Agnosia

Agnosia is the declining ability of the brain to interpret images transmitted by the eyes. The eyes do not actually "see"; they merely transmit images to the brain, which must then translate those images into something familiar or known. It is common for a person with Alzheimer's to be able to clearly and accurately describe her home, or a family member, but not be able to visually recognize her house or the family member who may be standing right in front of her.

A person with agnosia may not recognize a highway, road, train track, or environmental hazard, such as thorny bushes, thick underbrush or a body of water, and may well walk or drive into it. An Alzheimer's subject who still drives may not recognize a red light and drive into the intersection, or may not recognize a highway off-ramp as such, and enter a highway into oncoming traffic.

In addition, a person with agnosia may misunderstand a person's body language, facial expression, law enforcement uniform, or other visual cue as a threat, and react inappropriately or even violently.

Lastly, it is quite common for people with Alzheimer's to be encouraged to walk, maintain independence, or seek outdoor experiences. The loved one often agrees to a pattern of travel or behavior; i.e., "don't leave the house," "always stay within the neighborhood," or "don't cross Fifth Street." With such boundaries in place, caregivers often feel falsely secure.

Apraxia

Apraxia is the loss or reduction of the ability to coordinate fine and gross motor skills. For someone with Alzheimer's disease this may result in a change in gait or locomotor patterns.

Searchers should be aware that although a person may be a strong walker, over time or if forced to walk on soft surfaces, he will significantly tire, affecting his level of stress and symptoms.

Cognitive Mapping

Cognitive mapping is the brain's ability to memorize patterns and objects' locations. This ability makes it possible for a person to locate the bathroom in the middle of the night, with the lights off, use the toilet, and return to bed without requiring conscious thought.

Alzheimer's patients gradually lose this ability. This significantly hampers their ability to find their destinations or their way back home.

Lost and confused, it is common for wandering Alzheimer's patients to find a home, any home, and then attempt to enter it, particularly in developments in which many of the homes look alike.

Searchers should not rule out vacant homes in the area. Be alert for broken windows or locks, doors ajar, rifled gardens. Look for hoses that may have been left running, where someone has made an attempt to drink. Law enforcement in the area should be notified, and be alert for reports of returning homeowners who find something amiss.

Sundowning

Sundowning, or sundown syndrome, is agitation that typically occurs in the later hours of the day, often at sunset.

At this time, a person with dementia may experience an increase in confusion, agitation, aggression, paranoia, violence, obsessive behavior, and wandering. Significant decreases in physical capabilities, thinking, and speech, as well as other sensory deficits, also occur.

In essence, an Alzheimer's patient wandering during the late afternoon or early evening hours may be more agitated and afraid, and less rational, able to hear, see, or maintain his balance. He may not bunk down for the night, and instead push harder because of his altered perceptions. The result of this is often irrationally forging into areas such as dense brush, thick vegetation, or into hazardous terrain until he can go no further. He is less likely to respond to searchers who shout, call, or try to approach him. He may often purposely evade or hide from search teams.

When a subject is found, the risk of violence is usually highest during this period.

Elopement

Elopement is a form of wandering, common to Alzheimer's disease, that results in one's leaving the safety of the home, unable or unwilling to return. It can occur at any stage of the disease—early, middle or late.

> Sixty percent of people with Alzheimer's or a related dementia wander away from home and become lost at least once during the course of their disease.
>
> Once a person with Alzheimer's wanders away from home, 72% wander away again.[5]

A Life or Death Event

> *"911...what is your emergency?"*
>
> *"My mother is gone! She has Alzheimer's disease and wandered away." The voice is frantic. "Please, send someone quickly!"*

Every day across the United States, this scenario is played, and re-played, by law enforcement officers and search and rescue teams who respond to reports of missing Alzheimer's persons. Yet, while this type of call has become more and more commonplace, many persons underestimate the danger that a wandering Alzheimer's person faces.[6]

> If a wandering Alzheimer's patient is not found within 24 hours, he has only a 54% chance of survival.[7]

---

5. R. J. Koester and D. E. Stooksbury, "Lost Alzheimer's Subjects—Profiles and Statistics," *Response* 11(4) (1992): 20–26.
6. Kimberly R. Kelly Falconer, Search-and-Rescue volunteer with the San Diego County Sheriff's Department, Project Far From Home, www.projectfarfromhome.org.
7. R. J. Koester and D. E. Stooksbury, "Behavioral Profile of Possible Alzheimer's Disease Subjects in Search and Rescue Incidents in Virginia," *Wilderness and Environmental Medicine* 6 (1995): 34–43.

When a loved one (LO) disappears, time is critical. The sooner you can find him, the sooner you can remove him from the dangers that the "outside" world presents to a helpless victim of Alzheimer's disease. By providing clues to his intentions and mindset, the time and effort you put into reading and completing this workbook could save your loved one's life.

A wandering person with Alzheimer's is at the mercy not only of society, but also of the elements and basic rules of safety that we all take for granted. It cannot and should not be assumed that he can distinguish right from wrong; safe from unsafe; appropriate from inappropriate; nor be able to react to or protect himself from danger or injury.

- Not seeing or recognizing the danger of traffic, why not walk into a busy intersection?

- Not realizing that some people are ill-intentioned and may take advantage of him, why not approach a stranger?

- Not knowing that the home he seeks is 150 miles away and of a time long ago, why not head out and down the country road towards "home"?

- Not realizing the consequences of a frigid winter night, why put on a warm coat, robe, or even slippers—before heading out at 4:00 AM?

- Not realizing that the oncoming train cannot stop or turn to avoid him, why bother to step aside?

Causes of Elopement

All elopement is unintentional—at least in the sense that if the person were not cognitively impaired she would not be in danger of losing her way or fleeing from the safety of her home. However, the original reason for leaving may be either intentional or unintentional—the end result remaining the same: a person with Alzheimer's lost and unable to find her way back.

When a person with AD is intent upon escaping, going somewhere or finding someone/something, *she is on a mission.* There may be little that can be done to effectively discourage, distract or divert her. Once "the red flag is waved," the person should be very carefully supervised. And even if she forgets her desire for the moment, it should not be assumed that whatever triggered the intent will not do so again.

A person may *intentionally* elope for various reasons, including:

- Fleeing from a perceived threat, perpetrator or fear (paranoia, delusion or hallucination);

- Looking for a caregiver (who is simply out of sight);

- Attempting to once again go to work, school, etc. (retrogenesis);

- Seeking a person or destination that is real or from her past (alive or deceased), such as a spouse, son/daughter, mother/father, etc. (retrogenesis);

- Performing a former work task (such as distributing the mail, visiting a patient, a delivery route, etc.) (retrogenesis);

- Attempting to escape from pain, discomfort or too much environmental stimulation (people, activity, noises, etc.);

- Attempts to go "home" (although she actually was at home already) (retrogenesis);

- Going on a trip or moving, then seeking the former residence;

- Leaving home in anger, then not being able to find her way back.

With declining short-term memory, the person is less likely to be able to recall the events that led to her situation. Figuring out how she got to where she is, recalling the events that led her there, or retracing her path is impossible—the pieces of the puzzle are just not there.

> *"It's not where I'm going that is so difficult, it's how I got here."*
> *—An Alzheimer's patient*

But in many cases elopement is unintentional; that is, the person did not intend to leave her home or lose her way. She just suddenly found herself in an unfamiliar setting or situation and now "wanders" lost and confused, hopelessly seeking a way back or something familiar.

Causes of *unintentional* elopement include:

- Walking through or out of an exit door, perhaps mistaking it for the bathroom or kitchen door;

- Walking outside and not being able to recognize the house (or door) that she just exited;

- Becoming lost while taking a walk (even if she takes this walk every day, along the same route);

- Going on a short errand and becoming lost;

- Becoming overwhelmed by too much information, such as losing one's sense of direction in a crowd of people;

- Taking a shortcut and becoming lost;

- Getting caught outside after dark and becoming confused;

- Becoming lost while driving;

- Medication side effects;

- Walking to relieve pain or discomfort and becoming lost.

Wandering is not limited to just *walking* away. Loved ones can also become lost while driving. They can forget the way back home, fail to recognize where they are (thus not know how to return), forget where they intended to go (and just keep on driving) or have an accident (caused perhaps by mistaking the gas for the brake or failing to react to a situation quickly enough) and simply walk away—and away and away. These are all common forms of wandering that occur in a vehicle, rather than on foot.

"Some AD patients have driven hundreds and even thousands of miles from their homes. Others become disoriented while traveling out of town or around the local mall."[8]

Your loved one can also hitchhike, hail a cab, take a bus, or even test drive a new/used car. She doesn't have to be on foot to wander away from home. People in wheelchairs wander away from home, too.

Other Points to Consider

- It's not just people with Alzheimer's disease who may wander. People with any one of a number of diseases or conditions can also wander away from the safety of their home, unable or unwilling to return. These conditions include:

Parkinson's disease	Cognitive loss	Huntington's disease
Multiple strokes	Traumatic brain injury	Binswanger disease
Memory loss	Frontal-temporal dementia	Lewy Body disease
HIV dementia	Creutzfeldt-Jakob disease	Pick's disease
Progressive supranuclear palsy	Multi-infarct dementia	Vascular dementia
Alcohol-related dementia		

- A person does not have to be in the middle or late stages of Alzheimer's disease to become lost. Many cases involve people in the early stages of the disease.

- When one person elopes from a nursing home or assisted living facility, it should not be assumed that he did not leave with a friend or that others did not also follow him out the door.

Warning Signs of Potential Elopement

There's no way to predict who will wander, or when or how it might happen. Yet there are signs, hints or clues that might indicate that your loved one is looking for a way out or may soon become lost and unable to find his way home.

- Previous attempts to elope (once a person with Alzheimer's leaves home, it is likely that he will attempt to do so again);

- Repeated requests to go "home," or statements such as "I want to go home" (though the person may already be at home);

- Recurrent requests to go somewhere, or getting dressed to go to work, school, church, etc.;

---

8. C. E. Barber and D. Martin, *Alzheimer's Disease,* www.ext.colostate.edu/pubs/consumer/10233.html.

- Preparing to go to a location or an event (real or otherwise);

- Failure to realize that where he lives is his home;

- Failure to recognize the outside of his home or (once outside) how to get back inside;

- Failure to realize when he is lost;

- Increased episodes of disorientation;

- Sleep disorders, changes in sleep patterns or nocturnal wandering around the house;

- Concerns that involve a place outside of the home (to where he may feel the need to go, return, flee or seek refuge);

- Repeated recollections of earlier life events involving clandestine meetings (for example, running off to meet a boy or girlfriend or to a secret place where he played as a child);

- Packing a briefcase, suitcase or other accessory suggestive of a trip or going to work;

- Setting out for walks or errands and then forgetting where he was going;

- Delusions of people or events occurring in the home worthy of fleeing (e.g., strangers coming into the home with bad intentions, fear of being harmed if he remains at home, etc.);

- Inability to recognize the spouse or caregiver;

- Becoming lost in one's own home or having difficulty finding particular rooms;

- Confusion with regard to time or place that might suggest evasive or unusual behavior (such as believing one is overseas again during wartime);

- Returning from walks or drives later than usual or taking disproportionately long amounts of time to complete the trip;

- Inability to recognize otherwise familiar people, places and objects;

- Increased pacing or restlessness;

- Increased depression, agitation, anxiety, or panic attacks;

- Boredom or excess energy;

- Hallucinations, delusions or episodes of paranoia;

- Elevated concern when his caregiver or others are not within view;

- Repeated efforts to unlock gate or door locks or attempts to exit the yard;

- Confusing daytime and nighttime;

- Inability to distinguish dreams from reality;

- Repeated episodes of circling blocks or locations while driving in an attempt to find an address or destination.

How to Use This Workbook

This book is meant to be a workbook, designed to be filled out carefully and with thought—long before it is ever, if ever, needed. Take your time, think about the questions, and add or modify information as you think of it or as it changes.

In times of crisis we don't always think as clearly as we would like. Chaos, fear and trauma cause people to forget even the most common, everyday facts. It is far better to have this information written down, all in one place, allowing you to refer to it or maybe even just place it in the hands of law enforcement personnel during your time of need.

But most importantly, *In Search of the Alzheimer's Wanderer* is a tool to:

- identify, compile and make available important, potentially life-saving information;

- maximize the likelihood of finding a missing person with Alzheimer's;

- provide valuable information to help calm and communicate with your loved one once he is found; and

- help law enforcement personnel better understand your loved one and the unique demands that his condition imposes.

Though this workbook suggests that by striving to know the intent or destination of the wanderer you increase the chances of finding him, there are certainly no guarantees. No assumptions can or should be made; and no search should be solely directed to any one location or direction. Sometimes the person with Alzheimer's has an itinerary that we on the "outside" have no way of knowing. You and even the experts can only do the best you can with what you have available. That said, taking the right steps as soon as possible greatly increases the odds of finding a lost loved one.

Who Should Fill Out This Workbook?

There are three possible answers to this question:

- **Caregiving Team:** The caregiver, spouse, family member, friend, geriatric care manager, social worker, nursing home/small group home staff responsible for caring for your loved one with Alzheimer's disease; or

- **Family:** The spouse, family member, or friend *AND* the person with AD. This can be done as a team effort; or

- **Individual:** The person with AD himself. In many cases people experiencing memory loss, in the early stages of Alzheimer's disease, or who have just received a diagnosis of AD may want to begin providing information about themselves for their family, if and when one day the disease progresses to a point where they find themselves lost and in need of help. In such a case, this workbook might provide a tool or window to valuable information, provided by the actual victim of the disease.

Answer as many questions as possible. Though some of the questions in this workbook may seem silly or of little value, their answers may provide very important clues to trained law enforcement personnel. Answer every question that's applicable, no matter how unreasonable it may seem. You never know when that one answer will be the one bit of information that solves the mystery and brings your loved one home.

Whenever there is not enough space for all information or answers, feel free to insert a sheet of paper and keep it in the workbook, or add the information in blank spaces at the end of each section.

Not all questions may need to be answered. Some may not apply to you or your loved one. And some questions simply do not have answers—just leave them blank and go on to the next one. If you think of something later, you can always come back to it.

Take your time. Yes, there are a lot of questions, but completing this workbook does not have to be done all at once—take it one step at a time. Spend a half-hour today, then a half-hour tomorrow. In just a few days you'll be finished and your loved one safer.

Go ahead and get started. Don't procrastinate and don't set the workbook aside, promising to complete it later. Often the first step to any project is the toughest, so please sit down and just begin. I promise you, it will not be as difficult as you think—these are easy questions about the person whom you know the best.

Use a pencil, rather than a pen. When you fill out the forms, you'll want to use a pencil, rather than a pen. As things change, so do many of the answers. You'll want to make it as easy as possible for this information to be kept up-to-date and accurate. So if you need to correct something, change your mind or add information—make it easy for yourself!

Keep this workbook in a safe and familiar location. Ask yourself, "If there ever was an emergency, where would I look for this workbook?" Would it be in your desk drawer, kitchen drawer, or on a bookshelf? Then keep it there. (That is also why the workbook's cover is red—to make it easier to see and find in an emergency.)

Take photographs of your loved one. One should feature your loved one's face (taken from the shoulders up) and another of his full body, standing.

Have copies of the photos made (a minimum of 5 each) and attach a sticker on the back with your loved one's name and address, and your home and cell phone number. Do not write on the back of the photo, as the impression may transfer to the front and affect its duplication.

PHOTO TIPS

- Photos should be taken with your loved one wearing her favorite clothes and holding items that she likes to carry with her, such as a cane or purse.

- Take pictures with and without:
    Glasses
    Dentures
    Wigs or hairpieces

- In the close-up photo, your loved one should not be smiling. If she is lost, she probably won't be smiling.

- Update your photos every 6 months.

- Take photos of your loved one's favorite, or most often worn, pieces of clothing, and shoes, including the soles. Record her shoe size, and any identifying wear patterns. If she should ever wander, this will help trackers immensely.

Plan on sharing this workbook with law enforcement, search and rescue, and fire rescue personnel. This is not your personal phone book, nor is it a place to keep private information. It's a tool to find and return your loved one safely home, if one day she is discovered missing.

Update the workbook frequently. This workbook should be reviewed and updated frequently—as often as once a month would not be unreasonable. (Note that in the top right corner of many sections there is a place to fill in the last update.) Updating the book periodically will not only help you keep the information current, but also serve as a reminder to help you find the book in the event that you need to put your hands on it in a hurry.

> **The more often you review and update this workbook, the more
> likely it will be that all important bits of information will
> come to mind and be included.**

Some answers may also be time-sensitive or change as the disease progresses. Alzheimer's is a progressive disease, and as it advances people change, showing new interests and new perceptions of people, places and things in their life.

Store additional information in the workbook. We have provided a stick-on pocket with this book, which you may attach to either of the inside covers. This is a great way to store *copies* (not originals) of important items, papers and other information, making them immediately available if and when they are ever needed, including:

- ❏ Documentation of Power of Attorney
- ❏ Documentation of Legal Guardianship
- ❏ DNR (Do Not Resuscitate) Order
- ❏ Credit cards (copies with expiration date blacked out)

- ❏ Social Security card
- ❏ Health Insurance card
- ❏ Medical Information Release Forms

Multiple residences. If there is a summer and winter home or multiple residences, it would be advisable to have and fill out a workbook for each location (and keep it there). For additional copies call The Alzheimer's Store at (800) 752-3238.

This workbook is not cast in stone. Make modifications, adaptations, changes, and comments based on your particular situation and loved one. Remember, *everyone is different.*

One final note. Though primarily designed to assist in finding a lost loved one with Alzheimer's disease, many of the questions in this workbook are also designed to help first responders communicate and interact with your loved one once he is found—based on his condition, unique fears/concerns, and ways that will not further upset or confuse him. These include questions about his favorite topics of conversation, nicknames of familiar people, and behaviors that may possibly trouble your loved one.

> *It is our sincere wish that you will never need to put this workbook into action. But should your loved one ever wander away from the safety of his home and family, we hope that it becomes an integral tool leading to his safe and quick return.*
>
> *Please let us know of situations when this book has helped you or your loved one. Email us at AgelessD@aol.com. Please let us know if you have suggestions for future editions of* In Search of the Alzheimer's Wanderer.
>
> *Refer also to the* In Search of the Alzheimer's Wanderer *website:* www.alzwanderer.com.

Part 1

When a Loved One Is Missing

When a Loved One Is Missing

Last Updated: _____

When a loved one with Alzheimer's disease is discovered missing there are specific steps that should be taken and mistakes to be avoided. These are trying times, when even the best of us do not think as clearly as we would like. During such times, it is not unusual for a family member or caregiver to be so upset as to forget something as simple as their loved one's name.

The following sections are intended to help guide you through these steps, should you find yourself in such a situation, and highlight information that will help law enforcement find your loved one.

STEP ONE: Search Your Home
Needless to say, the first step is to conduct a thorough search of your home, critical areas of danger (pool, stairways, etc.) and immediate surroundings. See pages 82–83 and page 87 for more suggestions and details.

STEP TWO: Call 911
After conducting a thorough search of your home, you'll need to call the Police or Sheriff's Department (911) and provide them with some basic information. *Remember: Every minute counts, don't procrastinate!* (See page 23 for Steps 3 and 4.)

Once your loved one is discovered missing,

DO NOT WAIT MORE THAN 15 MINUTES BEFORE YOU CALL 911.

Basic information
What to tell the police or sheriff's department in the initial (911) phone call

Advise them that your loved one has Alzheimer's disease (or a related dementia) and that his/her disappearance is not voluntary.

(Many states now have a law that allows law enforcement to waive the 24-hour waiting period to report **missing, at risk, medically endangered elders.**)

Name of Loved One: _____ Age: _____

Male/Female: M ____   F ____ Height: ____ ft. ____ in.   Weight: _____ lbs.

Date of Birth ____ /____ /____   Complexion: Fair ____   Medium ____   Dark ____

Social Security No. _____   Race or Ethnicity _____

Describe loved one's body shape (thin, average, heavy, well-built, etc.) and any unique features.

_____

WHEN was your loved one last seen? Date ____/____/____   Day _____   Time _____

WHERE was your loved one last seen? _____

What was your loved one wearing? (See page 20) _____

_____

_____

YOUR Name _____ Relationship _____

Phone No. _____ Cell Phone No. _____

Is there a familiar name that your loved one uses to refer to you? _____

_____

(Loved One's) Current Home Address _____

Street, Unit/Apt. # _____

City _____ State _____ Zip _____

Tel. (_____) _____ How long has LO lived at this address? _____ yrs.

Who else lives with your loved one?

Name _____ Relationship _____

Sometimes the spouse or person living with your loved one is not the caregiver or a primary contact. It should be noted, in such cases, that there may be conditions important for law enforcement to know with regard to such people. For example, do they have dementia also? Are they someone with whom messages should not be left or who cannot be relied on to forward important information or to take certain actions?

Does this person have dementia?   Yes ____   No ____   Just Slightly ____

If this person answers the phone or door would a person assume or feel that he could speak to him/her about search results or actions needed to be taken?   Yes ____   No ____

If he/she answers the phone, should the caller ask to speak to someone else?

Yes ____   No ____   Who? _____

Can this person be relied on to act on or forward important information?   Yes ____   No ____

Does this person drive?   Yes ____   No ____

Is this person safe alone at home by him/herself?   Yes ____   No ____

Is this person at risk of leaving the house and endangering him/herself?   Yes ____   No ____

What was your loved one last wearing? (Include undergarments—shirt, blouse, T-shirt, etc.—as well, since a coat or outer garment might be discarded.)

Item	Size	Color/Style	Description
Hat/Cap/Head Scarf			
Shirt/Blouse			
T-Shirt/Undershirt			
Pants, Dress or Skirt			
Jump Suit/Warm-up Suit			
Sweater			
Robe			
Coat/Jacket			
Rain Gear			
Vest			
Tie/Neck Scarf			
Nightgown or Pajamas			
Shoes/Boots/Slippers			
Socks/Hose			
Underwear			
Belt			
Suspenders			
Gloves			
Necklace			
Earrings			
Bracelet			
Watch			
Safe Return or Wander ID Jewelry			
Other Jewelry			
Adult Brief			
Hearing Aid			
Dentures			
Wig/Hairpiece			

What items might your loved one be carrying (or have in pockets, purse, etc.)?

Things loved one collects _____

Tobacco products _____

Lighter, pocket knife, etc. _____

Purse or shopping bag _____

Wallet _____

Glasses/Sunglasses _____

Money _____

Cane/Walking Stick _____

Umbrella _____

Other: _____

_____

_____

What items might your loved one be carrying that she could drop, lose or discard (dentures, glasses, cap, etc.)?

_____

_____

_____

Does your loved one carry a purse or wallet? Yes _____   No _____   Does it have any features that make it unique (monogram, embroidery, phrases or images, names of people, places or companies)? If applicable, include a photo of it in the workbook.

Describe it _____

_____

What does she carry in it? (include all cards, even those which may be expired)

❏ Driver's License   ❏ Voter's Registration   ❏ _____ Credit Card*

❏ Car Insurance   ❏ Social Security   ❏ _____ Credit Card*

❏ Health Insurance   ❏ Car Registration   ❏ Library Card _____

❏ ATM Card   ❏ Keys   ❏ Other (Kleenex, candy, gum, matches)

❏ ID Card

Does your loved one carry a fanny pack, shopping bag or something else to carry "valuables"?

   Yes _____   No _____   Explain _____

*If you include your loved one's credit card number or a photocopy of the card, **do not include the expiration date.**

What items might your loved one be carrying *(continued)*

Miscellaneous membership cards:

❑ AAA   ❑ AARP   ❑ Photo (person in photo) _____

❑ Club _____   ❑ Photo (person in photo) _____

Does your loved one carry an Emergency Information (ID) card in her wallet or purse? Yes ____   No ____

Is all the information current and up to date? Yes ____   No ____

Are there ID labels sewn or ironed onto your loved one's clothing? Yes ____   No ____

Does your loved one carry a cell phone? Yes ____   No ____

If so, what is the cell phone number? (_____) _____

Does it have a GPS locator feature? Yes ____   No ____

Cell phone company name _____ Tel. No. (_____) _____

What else is missing?

❑ pet's leash	❑ car	❑ favorite article of clothing
❑ firearms	❑ pet	❑ suitcase
❑ wallet or purse	❑ bathrobe	❑ keys
❑ umbrella	❑ walker or wheelchair	❑ cash
❑ pocket knife	❑ motorized scooter	❑ riding lawnmower
❑ medications	❑ children*	❑ housekeeper or caregiver*
❑ other friends or family members*	❑ a neighbor's or visiting friend's car	❑ other residents (in nursing homes & ALFs)
❑ bicycle (color & type) _____	❑ other _____	❑ other _____

* This is not to suggest that anyone was taken against his will. Perhaps your loved one just went for a walk accompanied by another person. Provide a complete description of this person to law enforcement, if appropriate.

STEP THREE: Stay at Home and Wait for Law Enforcement Personnel to Arrive

STEP FOUR: The Initial Interview
Within a few minutes of reporting a missing person, law enforcement personnel should arrive at your door to conduct an initial interview. They will ask you a number of questions designed to collect specific information and to learn more about your missing loved one.

This information is critical to the success of the search. Completing this workbook before an incident occurs allows the search to begin sooner and equips the searchers with important information to help find your loved one.

The following pages will help you answer these questions and perhaps offer some suggestions as to additional information that may help in the search.

Investigating officers

❑ Police   ❑ Sheriff's Department   ❑ Detective (Unit) _____

❑ Fire/Rescue   ❑ Forest Service   ❑ Other _____

Name/Rank/Title	Telephone No.	Cell Phone No.

Fax number where information can be faxed to law enforcement (_____) _____

Case Number _____

NOTES

_____

_____

_____

_____

_____

_____

_____

_____

_____

_____

_____

_____

_____

_____

_____

_____

_____

_____

_____

_____

Questions to ask at the time of disappearance *(be prepared to answer when law enforcement personnel arrive)*

There are many questions in this workbook that may suggest potential destinations that your loved one may have in mind; however, where do *you* think your loved one might be headed?

- Is there anyone (a friend, caregiver, neighbor or relative) whom you have not been able to contact with regard to the whereabouts of your loved one? (Your loved one may be with that person.)
- When do you believe your loved one left home (i.e., how long has he been gone)?
- Was your loved one wearing any type of trackable wander alert bracelet or transmitter when last seen? (See pages 101–102 for more information on wander-alert devices.)
- Was he wearing a Safe Return or other Wander ID bracelet or necklace? (See pages 124–125 for more information on these programs.)

- Could he have left during the night? What time?
- Whom was he with when last seen (if anyone)? How can police contact this person?
- Who discovered him missing?

- Describe your loved one's general appearance when last seen. (Was he dressed as if ready to go to an event or did he more resemble a homeless person?)
- Might there be anything unusual about his appearance, such as underwear worn on the outside of his clothing, clothing inappropriate for seasonal conditions or social acceptance (indecent exposure)?
- Is he carrying identification or wearing any clothing labels that would provide his current address and/or telephone number?
- For men, when did he or was he last shaved? When did he have his last haircut?

- Was he wearing day or nighttime attire (pajamas/night gown, pants/shirt, jump suit, etc.)?
- Were his clothes clean or spotted from his last meal, etc.?
- Based on the season and climatic conditions, how likely or unlikely is it that your loved one is dressed appropriately?
- Could he be barefoot?
- Is he carrying anything with him that might seem unusual or out of the ordinary?

- What issues were recently on his mind (providing clues to where he might want to go)?
- What kinds of things has he been complaining about lately?
- Have there been any recent upsets? When? What about?
- Is there something that might have angered or frightened your loved one recently?
- Has he been talking about his childhood, past friends, deceased people in his life, work, school, parents, etc.?
- Have there been any events taking place in your neighborhood that might have attracted your loved one (such as school sporting events, parties, garage sales, etc.)?
- Has your loved one expressed seeing or hearing people, sounds, etc., that were not real?
- Were these events threatening or frightening to your loved one?

- Which door do you believe he went out (suggests a possible direction of travel)?
- Are there any familiar short-cuts (through woods, for example, or between buildings) that your loved one might have taken?
- Was your loved one's bed made this morning? Does he typically make his bed in the morning? Is he able to make his bed?
- What were the circumstances just before your loved one was discovered missing or when you last interacted with him?

- Does your loved one carry money, credit cards or an ATM card with him?
- How much cash would he have? (This might suggest how far he could get if taking public transportation.)
- Does he know his ATM PIN number?
- Does he know how to use an ATM machine or might he go to a bank to ask for money?
- Might he ask someone to help him?
- Would he know how to use a pay telephone to call you?

- Would your loved one try to hide from people searching for him?
- When your loved one is found, would he resist accompanying rescue personnel?
- Are there places other than home that your loved one might wish to be taken (somewhere that personnel can tell your loved one they are taking him to calm or appease him)?
- Does your loved one know to avoid traffic or how to cross streets safely?
- Does he recognize and react appropriately to dangerous situations?
- Does he overreact or panic easily?

- Are there any firearms kept in the house?
- Are they all accounted for? (Describe weapons if missing.)
- Are they kept loaded?
- Is ammunition stored nearby? Is all ammunition accounted for or is there ammunition missing?
- Does your loved one typically carry any other type of weapon, such as a knife?
- Would he use a weapon to defend himself?

- Was your loved one ever a boxer, martial artist or skilled in self-defense?
- How likely would your loved one be to use such skills if apprehended, discovered or cornered?
- Has your loved one been violent or physically abusive to you or others?
- Was your loved one ever a hiker, hunter or skilled in survival techniques?

- Is your car missing?
- When was the last time you filled the tank with gas?

Questions to ask at the time of disappearance *(continued)*

- How much gas do you estimate was in the car (full tank, three-quarters full, half a tank, one-quarter of a tank, or near empty)?
- Are all vehicles accounted for, including bicycles, riding lawnmowers, golf carts, etc.?
- If your loved one wears a hearing aid, was he wearing it when last seen? (Would he hear people calling for him or be able to respond to sounds, such as traffic?)
- When did your loved one eat last? Would he know how or where to get a meal when hungry?
- When did he bathe last?
- When were medications last given? When is the next time medications need to be given?
- What are the consequences of your loved one not taking his medications on time?

- If your loved one intended to go to "work," "school," "home," etc., where might he go?
- Have there been any events occurring in the neighborhood that might have upset your loved one or rekindled past concerns, such as neighborhood parties, robberies, sounds that resembled gunfire (e.g., fireworks or automobile backfires), etc.?
- Are there any current events or family affairs that your loved one has mentioned recently or showed concern about (such as a son/daughter's wedding or going to see a Veteran's Day parade (whether or not Veteran's Day is near)?
- Prior to your loved one's disappearance, were you, another family member or a caregiver away from the house? Where might your loved one have gone if he were looking for them?

NOTES

_____

_____

_____

_____

_____

_____

_____

_____

_____

_____

_____

_____

About Your Loved One

About Your Loved One

Full Name _____

Familiar Name/Nickname _____

Nickname that he/she was called as a child _____

Maiden Name(s) _____ , _____

Mother's Name _____ Still living? Yes ___ No ___

If deceased, when did she die? _____

Father's Name _____ Still living? Yes ___ No ___

If deceased, when did he die? _____

Physical Characteristics   Last Updated: _____

Describe your loved one's PHYSICAL condition:

❑ Excellent   ❑ Pretty Good   ❑ Good   ❑ Not Very Good   ❑ Poor

What words describe your loved one's appearance (tall, short, fat, skinny, buxom, petite, elderly, healthy, sickly, suntanned, pale, frail, etc.)? _____

_____

What would you say is your loved one's most distinguishing feature (bald, big nose, white hair, stooping, etc.)? _____

How do people describe your loved one? _____

_____

Does your loved one look like any famous or well-known person? Yes ___ No ___

  Who? _____

Does your loved one appear to be younger or older than his/her actual age? (Explain)

_____

_____

Birthmarks (include photo(s) and store them in the workbook)   Location _____

  Description: _____

Scars (include photo/s and store them in the workbook)   Location _____

  Description: _____

Tattoos (include photo/s and store them in the workbook)   Location _____

  Description: _____

Moles (include photo/s and store them in the workbook)   Location _____

Description: _____

Bruises or Recent Injuries   Location _____

Description of injury: _____

How and when did it happen? _____

_____

Casts or Bandages   Location _____

Description of injury: _____

How and when did it happen? _____

_____

Is your loved one right-handed or left-handed?   ❑ Right   ❑ Left   ❑ Ambidextrous

Eye Color: ❑ black   ❑ brown   ❑ green
              ❑ maroon   ❑ pink   ❑ blue
              ❑ gray   ❑ hazel   ❑ multi-colored

Does your loved one have all of his teeth?   Yes ____   No ____

What condition are his teeth in? _____

Are some or any of his teeth missing? (Describe) _____

Would you describe your loved one's teeth as   ❑ white   ❑ yellow   ❑ discolored
(Include a photo showing your loved one's teeth, if they might be an identifying feature.)

Does he wear dentures?   Yes ____   No ____   Top ____   Bottom ____   Both ____

Is there any type of identification code on the dentures?   Yes ____   No ____   Code _____

Does your loved one wear a hearing aid?   Yes ____   No ____

              ❑ right ear   ❑ left ear   ❑ both ears

Describe your loved one's ability to hear without his hearing aid(s):

              ❑ good   ❑ poor   ❑ cannot hear at all

Does your loved one wear glasses? Describe them _____

Describe his ability to see without glasses. (Day) _____ (Night) _____

How is your loved one's peripheral vision?   Good ____   Fair ____   Poor ____

He pays NO attention to people or things that are not directly in front of him ____

Physical Characteristics *(continued)*   Last Updated: _____

Has your loved one ever had a stroke?   Yes ____   No ____

Were there residual effects (contraction, partial paralysis—arm, leg, or arm and leg)?

Describe: _____ (right or left side) _____

Does your loved one:
- ❏ fall or lose his balance on sloping surfaces
- ❏ frequently need/look for places to sit down
- ❏ change directions or destinations
- ❏ sway or meander (vs. walking in straight lines)
- ❏ vary gait (short and long steps)
- ❏ walk very slowly
- ❏ take short steps
- ❏ shuffle
- ❏ limp or drag one foot
- ❏ drag feet when walking

Yes ____   No ____   Sometimes ____   Explain _____

When necessary, can your loved one run or walk fast? Yes ____   No ____   Sometimes ____

Is your loved one at risk of falling if he attempts to walk unassisted?   Yes ____   No ____

Is there anything distinctive or unique about the way your loved one walks?   Yes ____   No ____

After short rests is your loved one able to walk without assistance?   Yes ____   No ____

Does your loved one use or require a walker ____ or cane ____ ?

   Sometimes ____ All of the time ____

Was your loved one ever a long-distance walker or hiker? Yes ____   No ____   When? _____

Is your loved one more apt to stay on roads or paths or possibly stray off-trail?

   (Explain) _____

Does your loved one use a wheelchair? Yes ____   No ____

Is he able to get out of his wheelchair and walk for short distances? Yes ____   No ____

   How far? _____

Is your loved one able to propel himself (or scoot) in his wheelchair?

   Yes ____   No ____   Explain _____

Did your loved one ever learn to swim? Yes ____   No ____

Can he/she still swim?   Yes ____   No ____   Just a little ____   I don't know ____

Hair: ❏ full head of hair   ❏ partial balding (front)   ❏ partial balding (rear spot)   ❏ mostly bald

   ❏ completely bald   ❏ hairpiece   ❏ receding hairline

Hair Color *(check all that apply)*:

❑ Black   ❑ Red/Auburn   ❑ Sandy   ❑ Gray   ❑ White

❑ Blonde/Strawberry   ❑ Brown   ❑ Partially Gray

Is your loved one's hair: ❑ Artificially colored   ❑ Natural

Hair Style Description: _____

❑ Does your loved one wear a hairpiece or wig? Yes ____   No ____

Description: _____

(Do you have a recent photo showing loved one's hair style? This would serve much better than a description.)

❑ Recent changes in hair length, color or style _____

Last time your loved one had his hair done or received a haircut: _____ days ago.

Facial Hair

❑ Mustache   ❑ Beard (full)   ❑ Goatee   ❑ Sideburns   ❑ Scruffy or Unshaven

Explain _____
(Do you have a recent photo showing loved one's facial hair style? This would serve much better than a description.)

What is your loved one's shoe size? _____

What type of shoe is he most likely to be wearing? _____

What brand of shoe? _____

Color: _____ Does it have a smooth or patterned sole? _____

Does your loved one wear orthopedic shoes? Yes ____   No ____   Color _____

Does your loved one have any noticeable physical abnormalities? Yes ____   No ____

Explain _____

Does your loved one have any missing limbs? If so, explain _____

Does your loved one have or use any artificial prosthesis? Yes ____   No ____

Describe _____

Does your loved one have any other disabilities or abnormalities not previously mentioned?

Yes ____   No ____   Explain _____

Daily Routines   Last Updated: _____

Does your loved one take daily walks? Yes ____   No ____   Approx. distance _____

Morning walk (time) _____ AM   Afternoon walk (time) _____ PM

Where does he typically go? *(Describe his route; use extra paper if necessary)*

Whom does he like to talk to along the way? _____

In what direction does he typically begin walking? _____

For how long is he typically gone? _____ (hours) _____ (minutes)

Is this the first time he has left home, failed to return on time, or gotten lost?

Yes ____   No ____   Number of times ____   Explain _____

_____

Is (or has been) walking a part of a daily routine, including walking to work, school, church, temple, etc.?

Yes ____   No ____   Explain _____

_____

Is he still able to walk for long distances? Yes ____   No ____   How far? _____

Is a bicycle ride, going to get the mail or newspaper, or other reason to travel outdoors part of your loved one's

daily routine? Yes ____   No ____

Does your loved one walk the family dog? Yes ____   No ____   Where? _____

_____ Color of leash _____

What are your loved one's sleep patterns? When does he typically wake up at night?

_____ PM, _____ PM, _____ AM, _____ AM, _____ AM

What does your loved one typically do when up and about at night? _____

_____

What time does your loved one like to get up in the morning? _____

What does he do when he gets up (morning routines)? _____

_____

Was meeting with anyone or spending time at any locale part of a daily or day-of-the-week routine (for example
something your loved one did on Tuesdays)? Yes ____   No ____

❑ At a bar   ❑ At a restaurant with friends   ❑ Going to church/temple   ❑ Visiting friends

❑ At a daycare facility   ❑ Other (Explain) _____

_____

Likes and Dislikes   Last Updated: _____

Does your loved one currently have a pet? Yes ____   No ____

Name _____ *(Store a picture of the pet in the workbook.)*

Type of animal: ❏ Dog   ❏ Cat   ❏ Other _____

Describe the pet's leash and collar _____

Would your loved one take the pet with him if he were to leave the house? Yes ____   No ____

Where might he take the pet if it were hurt or sick? _____

Did your loved one have a pet in the past? Yes ____   No ____

Pet's name _____ How long ago? _____

Type of animal: ❏ Dog   ❏ Cat   ❏ Other _____

Did your loved one have a pet as a child (that he recalls)? Yes ____   No ____

Name _____

Type of animal: ❏ Dog   ❏ Cat   ❏ Other _____

Does your loved one have a favorite place in the neighborhood where he likes to go?

❏ a school yard (to watch children)   ❏ a park bench   ❏ a campground   ❏ a pond or lake

❏ a park (describe favorite spot within the park)   ❏ fishing or boat dock

❏ other (Explain) _____

Does your loved one have a place in the neighborhood where he likes to go to be alone?

Yes ____   No ____   How often does he go there? _____

Where is it? _____

Is there a place in the neighborhood that your loved one frequented or played at as a child?

Explain _____

_____

Does your loved one like to take short walks or go walking in the woods? Yes ____   No ____

Does your loved one typically or routinely walk to any places in the neighborhood?

❏ drug store   ❏ barber shop   ❏ grocery store   ❏ doctor's office   ❏ beauty salon

❏ church or temple   ❏ neighbor's house   ❏ friend's house   ❏ local restaurant

❏ diner or coffee shop   ❏ ATM machine   ❏ bank   ❏ movie theater   ❏ mail box

❏ other _____

_____

Likes and Dislikes *(continued)*

Who are people in your neighborhood with whom your loved one interacts regularly?

❏ Postman/woman   ❏ Barber   ❏ Grocer   ❏ Pharmacist   ❏ Bank teller

❏ Diner waiter/waitress   ❏ Neighbor   ❏ Policeman/woman

❏ Children (playing or coming from or going to school)   ❏ Other _____

Explain (provide name(s)) _____

Does your loved one typically accompany you (or anyone else) when you go on errands?

Where? _____

What are your loved one's favorite pastimes and hobbies?

❏ fishing   ❏ yard work   ❏ crafts   ❏ gardening   ❏ cooking   ❏ walking

❏ people watching   ❏ church or temple   ❏ reading the newspaper   ❏ painting

❏ playing a musical instrument   ❏ feeding birds, etc.   ❏ sitting on the porch or in the backyard

❏ other _____

What hobbies or pastimes did your loved one have that he had to give up, perhaps due to the disease or other age-related condition? (For example: hunting, hiking, fishing, jogging, bicycle riding, etc.)

_____ , _____ , _____

Does your loved one have a favorite local restaurant? Yes ____ No ____

❏ IHOP   ❏ McDonald's/Burger King   ❏ Local Diner   ❏ Other

Explain _____

Who are respected authority figures for your loved one (people whose opinions are important and reliable to your loved one)?

❏ Police officers   ❏ Soldiers   ❏ Women   ❏ Nurses   ❏ Clergy

❏ Men   ❏ Teachers   ❏ Caregivers   ❏ People in uniform   ❏ Doctors

❏ Family members _____ , _____ , _____

❏ Other _____ Explain _____

Who among your friends, family or community are people whose instructions your loved one would follow? If their information is not already provided, please use an extra sheet of paper to add it.

Name	Relation

Favorite Things   Last Updated: _____

Complete this sentence:

"_____ (LO) would never leave the house without his/her _____."

(For example: shoes, cane/walking stick, hat, keys, glasses, pipe, checkbook, gloves, wallet, purse, cap, wig, jacket, favorite article of clothing, robe, jewelry, lipstick, compact)

Item	Description *(whenever possible, include photo of item)*

Does your loved one smoke cigarettes? Yes ____   No ____   Brand _____

Would your loved one approach a stranger to ask for a cigarette? Yes ____   No ____   Maybe ____

Favorite candy bar _____

Favorite snack _____

Does your loved one collect or habitually carry any items, such as sugar packets? (Explain)

_____

NOTES

_____

_____

_____

_____

_____

_____

_____

_____

_____

_____

_____

_____

_____

Life History

Last Updated: _____

Where was your loved one born? _____, _____ (city, state)

(country, if other than U.S.) _____

Where was your loved one raised (childhood)? _____, _____ (city, state)

(country, if other than U.S.) _____ Language spoken _____

Where did your loved one grow up (teen years)? _____, _____ (city, state)

(country, if other than U.S.) _____ Language spoken _____

Where did she live in the past (city, state)? (list most recent residences first)

_____ Approximate year left_____ Years lived there _____

_____ Approximate year left_____ Years lived there _____

_____ Approximate year left_____ Years lived there _____

_____ Approximate year left_____ Years lived there _____

What jobs or careers did your loved one have during her life? (most recent one first)

1. _____ Job responsibilities_____ ,

_____

2. _____ Job responsibilities_____ ,

_____

3. _____ Job responsibilities_____ ,

_____

Which job does she regard as her predominant career or trade? _____

What hours did she work? From _____ AM / PM to _____ AM / PM

What time did she typically leave home to go to work? _____ AM / PM

How did she get to work? _____

Was her office or work location near her home? Yes _____   No _____

When did she retire? _____

Does she believe she still lives close to her work (or school, etc.)? Yes _____   No _____

Does she ever mention going to work or still having a job? Yes _____   No _____

For women who were mothers or homemakers, what tasks were part of your loved one's daily routines (involving travel or driving)?   ❏ Caring for a spouse   ❏ Picking up children from school   ❏ Going home to prepare supper   ❏ Other _____

If your loved one were to try to help someone, what kinds of tasks might she most likely offer to do?

_____ , _____

Military Service   Last Updated: _____

In what branch of the military did your loved one serve (if applicable)?

❑ Army   ❑ Navy   ❑ Marines   ❑ Air Force   ❑ Coast Guard   ❑ None   ❑ Other

What were his responsibilities? _____

Where was he stationed? _____, _____

Did he serve during wartime? Yes _____ No _____ Which war? _____

Did he serve in the military service for another country? Yes _____ No _____

When: _____, _____ to _____, _____

Where: _____

What language did he speak in that service? _____

Was your loved one ever captured by the enemy, imprisoned, MIA or a POW?

Yes _____ No _____ What ethnicity/nationality were his captors? _____

Was he trained in survival? Yes _____ No _____

Does your loved one have flashbacks or relive events that occurred while he was in the service (e.g., delusions that people are enemy soldiers or fears of being caught by the enemy)? Yes _____ No _____

Explain _____

Does your loved one believe that he is still in the service? Yes _____ No _____

Explain (use extra paper if necessary) _____

_____

Does your loved one enjoy wearing any type of military apparel (e.g., hat identifying his service or ship, "dog tags")?

Yes _____ No _____ Describe (include a photo) _____

_____

Comments: Perhaps these questions brought to mind additional ideas or comments that you think might be helpful for rescue personnel to know. Here's a great place to note them.

_____

_____

_____

_____

_____

_____

_____

Dementia-Related Traits   Last Updated: _____

What stage of Alzheimer's would you say your loved one is in? (Check one)

❑ Early   ❑ Early/Middle   ❑ Middle   ❑ Middle/Late   ❑ Late

(See pages 3–4 for description of stages)

Most recent MMSE (Mini-Mental Status Exam) Score (obtain from physician) _____

Date tested _____

Does your loved one know her own name? Yes ____ No ____ Not all of the time ____

Is she able to tell a police officer or stranger what her name is? Yes ____ No ____

Even if your loved one says that she does not know her name, if asked to do so, can she WRITE her name?

Yes ____ No ____ Sometimes ____ (Ask her)

Does your loved one know her current telephone number? Yes ____ No ____

Even if your loved one says that she does not know her telephone number, if asked to do so, can she WRITE it?

Yes ____ No ____ Sometimes ____ (Ask her)

Is she able to tell someone where she lives? Yes ____ No ____ Sometimes ____

Does she know what city and state she lives in? Yes ____ No ____ Sometimes ____

If not, in what city and state does she believe she lives? _____ (Ask her)

Would your loved one ask a stranger for assistance to take her home?

Yes ____ No ____ Possibly ____ Unlikely ____

Does your loved one respond to her name? Yes ____ No ____ Not all of the time ____

To what other name might she respond? _____

How old does your loved one think she is? _____ (Ask her)

What year does she believe she was born? _____ (Ask her)

What year does she believe this is? _____ (Ask her)

Who does your loved one think is president? _____ (Ask her)

What world events does she believe are now taking place? (Ask her) _____

_____

Would your loved one attempt to use long-distance public transportation (taxi, bus, train, plane)?

Possibly ____   Unlikely ____   Impossible ____

Has she tried before? Yes ____ No ____ When? _____

How many times? _____ Where did she try to go? _____

If your loved one attempted to get to another location, what story might she tell a Good Samaritan to ask for assistance or to help her get there? (This might be something fictitious or a story that your loved one honestly believes to be true.)

_____

_____

What other stories has she used in the past? _____

_____

Does your loved one recognize her own reflection in a mirror? (Or does she think it might be another person?)

　Explain _____

Is your loved one able to hide her confusion (act normal) for short periods of time?   Yes _____   No _____

How capable of fooling someone would you say she is?

　❏ Not at all capable　　❏ Somewhat capable　　❏ Very capable

When frightened or upset, does your loved one seek people _____ or solitude_____?

Are there descriptions or phrases that your loved one uses to describe possible destinations?
(e.g., a former office = "the place where _____," a school = "the place where the little people go," a friend's house = "the blue house," etc.)

　Explain _____

_____

Destination	Address	LO's description of this location

Is there any behavior that your loved one may exhibit that might cause public attention or cause her to be arrested (disrobing or urinating in public, eating a meal or taking a product from a store without paying for it, becoming aggressive or loud, cursing at people, etc.)? Yes _____   No _____

Explain _____

_____

Medical Information   Last Updated: _____

Was an Alzheimer's diagnosis made?

Yes ____   No ____   Date of Alzheimer's diagnosis _____ / _____ / _____

Dr.'s Name _____ Dr.'s Tel. No. (_____) _____

City, state of doctor _____ Emergency Tel. No. (_____) _____

Name of family doctor _____ Dr.'s Tel. No. (_____) _____

City, state of doctor _____ Emergency Tel. No. (_____) _____

What type of dementia does your loved one have? *(Check all that apply)*

❑ Dementia of the Alzheimer's Type (DAT)   ❑ Parkinsonian dementia   ❑ Pick's Disease (FTD)

❑ Multi-infarct   ❑ Huntington's disease   ❑ Stroke   ❑ CJD   ❑ Binswanger disease

❑ Lewy Body   ❑ HIV dementia   ❑ You do not know, (it's just dementia)

❑ Other _____

Health Insurance Co. _____ Ins. Agent _____

Policy Number _____ Tel. No. (_____) _____

Make sure that you update this health insurance information if you have any company or policy changes.

Is there a DNR (Do Not Resuscitate) order filled out and filed for your loved one?

Yes ____   No ____   Where is it kept? _____
(Make a copy and keep it in this workbook)

Date of last Tetanus Shot _____ / _____ / _____   LO's Blood Type _____

Medicare No. _____ Medicaid No. _____

Preferred hospital if medical attention is required _____

NOTES

_____
_____
_____
_____
_____
_____
_____
_____

Other Medical Conditions   Last Updated: _____

List all other medical conditions that your loved one may have (use an extra piece of paper if necessary):

❏ Parkinson's	❏ Diabetes	❏ Heart condition
❏ Stroke	❏ Cancer	❏ Kidney condition (requiring dialysis)
❏ High blood pressure	❏ Asthma	❏ Epilepsy
❏ Breathing difficulties	❏ Angina	❏ Depression
❏ Visual impairment	❏ Deaf (completely)	❏ Paranoia
❏ Incontinence (urinary)	❏ Seizure disorder	❏ Alcoholism
❏ Incontinence (fecal)	❏ Blind (full, partial, right side, left side)	❏ Hearing loss/impairment

❏ Delusions or hallucinations   ❏ Bleeding or blood clot disorder

❏ Difficulty urinating   ❏ Colostomy or ileostomy

❏ Difficulty walking   ❏ Arthritis (explain) _____

❏ Osteoporosis—are there visible signs (such as a dowager's hump or stooping posture)?

    Yes ____   No ____   ❏ Other _____

    _____

Does your loved one have any allergies? Yes ____   No ____

    ❏ Foods _____   ❏ Insect stings/bites_____

    ❏ Medications _____   ❏ Other _____

Does he/she have severe allergic reactions to anything? Yes ____   No ____

    To what? _____

Does your loved one have any conditions or injuries that require monitoring or constant treatment (e.g., open wounds that do not heal, etc.?) Yes ____   No ____

    Explain _____

    _____

Does your loved one have difficulty swallowing? Yes ____   No ____

Do medications have to be ground up and mixed with food in order for your loved one to take them?

    Yes ____   No ____   Favorite food(s) to mix meds with _____

    _____

Does your loved one wear adult briefs? Yes ____   No ____   Size ____   Brand _____

    Type/Style (light/medium/heavy—panty, jockey short or boxer, etc.) _____

Other Medical Conditions *(continued)*

Surgeries that your loved one has had which left scars or visible evidence (check all that apply):

❏ Colostomy or Ileostomy   ❏ Amputation   ❏ Hernia   ❏ Pacemaker Insertion

❏ Appendectomy   ❏ Hysterectomy   ❏ Heart Surgery   ❏ Gall Bladder

❏ Mastectomy   ❏ Organ Transplant   ❏ Cosmetic Surgery   ❏ Cesarean section

❏ Other (Explain)

_____

_____

_____

_____

NOTES

_____

_____

_____

_____

_____

_____

_____

_____

_____

_____

_____

_____

_____

_____

_____

_____

_____

Prescription Drugs (loved one is currently taking)

Last Updated: _____

Critical Meds (✓)	Medication	Dosage	Taken for (condition)	Medication Times
				____ AM ____ PM
				____ AM ____ PM
				____ AM ____ PM
				____ AM ____ PM
				____ AM ____ PM
				____ AM ____ PM
				____ AM ____ PM
				____ AM ____ PM
				____ AM ____ PM
				____ AM ____ PM
				____ AM ____ PM

What ill effects might result from failure to take medications? Explain _____

_____

Where in the home are medications kept?

❏ Bathroom medicine cabinet   ❏ Kitchen cabinet/shelf   ❏ Kitchen counter   ❏ Refrigerator

❏ Kitchen/dining room table   ❏ Other _____

Where do you fill your prescriptions? *(This information can be found on the medicine bottles.)*

(Drug store or pharmacy) _____

Pharmacist's name _____ Telephone no. _____

Non-prescription (over-the-counter) products that your loved one may also be taking:

Non-Prescription Drugs/Herbs/Vitamins	Dosage	Taken for (condition)	When Taken
			____ AM ____ PM
			____ AM ____ PM

Prescription Drugs *(continued)*

Special instructions in case of a medical emergency:

_____

_____

_____

_____

_____

_____

_____

_____

NOTES

_____

_____

_____

_____

_____

_____

_____

_____

_____

_____

_____

_____

_____

_____

"Home"

Does your loved one know his current address?   Yes ____   No ____   Sometimes ____

Even if your loved one says that he does not know his address, if asked to do so, can he WRITE his address?

Yes ____   No ____   Sometimes ____   (Ask him)

How does your loved one describe his home (e.g., the "white" building, the place with green awnings, etc.)?

_____

_____

Where does your loved one call "home" (e.g., his actual home, a past home, his childhood home, the nursing home, the assisted living facility, etc.)?   Explain _____

_____

Could "home" refer to anywhere else?   Yes ____   No ____   Unlikely ____

Explain _____

Where does your loved one believe his home is (e.g., "on the other side of that hill," etc.)?

_____

Are there any nearby buildings or structures that resemble or remind your loved one of a former residence or place of work?

Yes ____   No ____   Explain _____

_____

Are there nearby homes, buildings, apartments or other units that resemble your loved one's residence?

Yes ____   No ____   Explain _____

_____

Alternate Home: (summer or winter home, for example)

Street _____ Unit/Apt. # _____

City _____ State ____ Zip _____

Tel. (_____) _____

Seasonal schedule (What times of the year are spent at each location?):

Alternate home: from _____ to _____

Current home: from _____ to _____

Is it possible that your loved one might ask a mass transit operator for assistance or instruct a cab driver to take him there?   Yes ____   No ____   Possibly ____   Unlikely ____

"**Home**" *(continued)*

Would your loved one ask a stranger for assistance to take him there?

 Yes ____   No ____   Possibly ____   Unlikely ____

How does your loved one describe his other home (e.g., the "white" building, the place with green awnings, etc.)?

_____

_____

_____

_____

Does anyone live there when you are not there? Yes ____   No ____

 Who? _____

Past Address #1: (Where did your loved one live before he moved to his current home?)

Name of family living there now: _____   Tel. No. _____

Street _____   Unit/Apt. # _____

City _____   State ____   Zip _____

When did your loved one live at this location? _____ to _____

Who lived there with him? _____   Relation _____

Does he remember this home? Yes ____   No ____   Sometimes ____

Does he talk about this home or offer any reason for trying to return there? Yes ____   No ____

How far away is it? _____ miles

Would your loved one try to go to this home? Likely ____   Unlikely ____   Possibly ____

Would he know how to get there? Yes ____   No ____   Possibly ____   Unlikely ____

What means of transportation would he most likely use to get there? _____

When was the last time he mentioned this home? _____

Is it possible that your loved one might ask a mass transit operator for assistance or instruct a cab driver to take him to this location?

 Yes ____   No ____   Likely ____   Unlikely ____   Explain _____

Would your loved one ask a stranger for assistance to take him there?

 Yes ____   No ____   Possibly ____   Unlikely ____

Past Address #2: (Include any and all addresses that remain familiar to your loved one—use extra sheets of paper if necessary)

Name of family living there now: _____ Tel. No. _____

Street _____ Unit/Apt. # _____

City _____ State _____ Zip _____

When did your loved one live at this residence? _____ to _____

Who lived there with him?_____

Does he remember this home? Yes _____   No _____

Does he talk about this home or offer any reason for trying to return there? Yes _____   No _____

How far away is it? _____ miles

Would your loved one try to go to this home? Likely _____   Unlikely _____   Possibly _____

Would he know how to get there? Yes _____   No _____   Possibly _____   Unlikely _____

What means of transportation would he most likely use to get there? _____

When was the last time he mentioned this home? _____

Is it possible that your loved one might ask a mass transit operator for assistance or instruct a cab driver to take him to this location?

  Yes _____   No _____   Likely _____   Unlikely _____   Explain _____

  _____

Would your loved one ask a stranger for assistance to take him there?

  Yes _____   No _____   Possibly _____   Unlikely _____

NOTES

_____

_____

_____

_____

_____

_____

_____

_____

_____

Medical Jewelry   Last Updated: _____

Does your loved one wear a Safe Return bracelet or necklace (or one from your local Alzheimer's organization)?

Yes ____   No ____

Bracelet ID Number _____ (This can be found on the back of the Safe Return bracelet.)

If your loved one's medical ID jewelry is from an organization other than the Alzheimer's Association Safe Return Program:

Organization _____

Telephone Number (_____) _____

(For more information on the Alzheimer's Association Safe Return Program see page 124.)

Does your loved one wear a Medic Alert bracelet ____ or necklace ____?   Yes ____   No ____

Medical Condition noted on bracelet _____

Does your loved one wear any type of TRACKABLE wander alert bracelet or transmitter?

Yes ____   No ____   (For more information about trackable wander alert devices see pages 102 and 142.)

Name of Company _____ Tel. No. (_____) _____

LO's ID # _____

NOTES

_____

_____

_____

_____

_____

_____

_____

_____

_____

_____

_____

_____

_____

_____

Wandering History Last Updated: _____

Does your loved one have a history of wandering? Yes ____ No ____

Number of attempts to leave home in the last 6 months _____, in the last year _____

When was the last attempt (successful or unsuccessful) to leave home? Day of week ____ Month _____ Year ____

Where did your loved one intend to go? _____

How recent was the last successful attempt to leave home? Day of week ____ Month _____ Year ____

Where did she want to go? _____

Where and how far away was she found? _____

_____

(Use an additional piece of paper to record any history of attempts to leave home and the details associated with each episode.)

How was she discovered? _____

Does or would your loved one attempt to drive? Yes ____ No ____ Possibly ____ Unlikely ____

Where might your loved one go on an errand?

❑ Post office   ❑ Bank or ATM   ❑ Liquor store   ❑ Drug store

❑ Grocery store   ❑ Walk the dog   ❑ Barber shop or beauty salon

❑ Newspaper stand ❑ convenience store, gas station or other nearby shopping mart

❑ Other _____

(Name, location, phone number) _____

_____

What modes of transportation can your loved one still use or attempt to use?

❑ Walk   ❑ Bus   ❑ Cab   ❑ Transit train

❑ Plane   ❑ Hitchhike   ❑ Accept a ride from a stranger   ❑ Family car

❑ Bicycle   ❑ Ask a neighbor or friend for a ride

❑ Other (Explain) _____

What type(s) of transportation does your loved one like/prefer to use?

❑ Walk   ❑ Bus   ❑ Cab   ❑ Transit train

❑ Plane   ❑ Hitchhike   ❑ Accept a ride from a stranger   ❑ Family car

❑ Bicycle   ❑ Ask a neighbor or friend for a ride

❑ Other (Explain) _____

Would your loved one attempt to rent, lease, test drive, or buy a car? Yes ____ No ____

Recent Behavior   Last Updated: _____

Has your loved one been demonstrating any unusual behaviors lately (disrobing in public, asking unusual questions, packing to go somewhere, dressing unusually, voicing anger or concerns regarding an individual whom he may attempt/need to visit, etc.)?

Explain _____

_____

_____

_____

_____

Have you observed any changes in your loved one's behaviors or habits lately?

Explain _____

_____

_____

_____

_____

Has your loved one been talking about any events that might suggest travel, such as:

- ❏ visiting a family member
- ❏ the birth of a grandchild
- ❏ going "home" or going to work
- ❏ going to school
- ❏ a family reunion
- ❏ attending a funeral
- ❏ a religious event
- ❏ visiting a friend
- ❏ a wedding
- ❏ a trip
- ❏ a graduation

❏ other (Explain) _____

Has your loved one been experiencing or mentioning any fears or concerns lately (for example, being placed in a nursing home)?

Yes ____   No ____   Explain: _____

_____

When your loved one is angry, does he speak of going anywhere special? Yes ____   No ____

Where? _____

What have been some of the subjects of recent delusions? (e.g., "People are coming into my house and stealing things," "chasing me," "stalking me," "watching me," "hurting me," "people are imprisoned here" (a nursing home, for example), etc.) _____

_____

_____

Has your loved one experienced any hallucinations recently? Yes ____ No ____

   Explain _____

What issues/concerns has your loved one been expressing lately? (e.g., Can't find deceased spouse, picking up his children from school, meeting past girlfriends, a pet he once had, etc.)

_____

_____

Have there been any recent changes in the home or family?

❏ loss of a pet	❏ renovations/redecorating	❏ new furniture
❏ new room assignments	❏ home additions	❏ loss of a family member
❏ absence of a family member	❏ a new child	❏ a new pet
❏ arguing or family disagreements	❏ change in daily routines	❏ rearranged furniture

❏ other _____

If there was a loss of a pet, is there another *similar* pet in the neighborhood that your loved one might have seen and mistaken for his lost pet? Yes ____ No ____

NOTES

_____

_____

_____

_____

_____

_____

_____

_____

_____

_____

_____

_____

_____

NOTES

Part 3

Important Information

Important Information

Last Updated: _____

The Family Car

We have: ❏ One family car ❏ Two family cars ❏ No family cars

Make of Car: _____ Model: _____

Year: _____ Lic. Plate # _____ License Plate State _____

Color(s): _____

Who is the registered owner of the car? _____

Do you have a personalized license plate?   Yes _____   No _____

Does your car have any unique features (such as tool boxes for pick-up trucks, antenna decorations, etc.)?

  Yes _____   No _____   Describe: _____

_____

Are there any bumper stickers or appliques on the back of the car?   Yes _____   No _____

  Describe them _____

Are there any noticeable dents, scratches or exterior parts visibly broken?   Yes _____   No _____

  Explain _____

How many sets of keys are there for this car? _____

Who keeps them? _____

Have any keys been lost lately? Yes _____   No _____   Were they found? Yes _____   No _____

Is your car equipped with LoJack, OnStar or other GPS locating device? Yes _____   No _____

  ID No. _____ Company Emergency Tel. No._____

Second Car

Make of Car: _____ Model: _____

Year: _____ Lic. Plate # _____ License Plate State _____

Color(s): _____

Who is the registered owner of the car? _____

Do you have a personalized license plate?   Yes _____   No _____

Does your car have any unique features (such as tool boxes for pick-up trucks, antenna decorations, etc.)?

  Yes _____   No _____   Describe: _____

_____

Are there any bumper stickers or appliques on the back of the car?   Yes _____   No _____

  Describe them _____

Are there any noticeable dents, scratches or exterior parts visibly broken?   Yes _____   No _____

  Explain _____

How many sets of keys are there for this car? _____

Who keeps them? _____

Have any keys been lost lately? Yes _____   No _____   Were they found? Yes _____   No _____

Is your car equipped with LoJack, OnStar or other GPS locating device? Yes _____   No _____

  ID No. _____ Company Emergency Tel. No._____

NOTES

_____
_____
_____
_____
_____
_____
_____
_____
_____
_____
_____
_____
_____
_____
_____
_____
_____
_____
_____

The Neighborhood

Last Updated: _____

Do you or a close neighbor have a swimming pool?   Yes ____   No ____

Do you live in a gated community (Is there a 24-hour monitored gatehouse)?   Yes ____   No ____

List immediate dangers in your neighborhood.

❏ Railroad tracks	❏ Rivers	❏ Lake, pond, or river
❏ Highway overpasses	❏ Desert	❏ Woods
❏ Bridges	❏ Caves or mines	❏ Drainage canals
❏ Tunnels	❏ Industrial areas	❏ Mountains or cliffs
❏ Swamps	❏ Culverts	❏ Steep paths or stairways
❏ Vast crop fields	❏ Cattle yards or pens	❏ Dangerous urban areas
❏ Construction sites	❏ Cliffs or steep embankments	❏ Fishing or boat docks
❏ Busy intersections	❏ Highways or high traffic streets	❏ Garbage dumpsters
❏ Golf course (with water traps)	❏ Wrecked or abandoned vehicles	❏ Abandoned buildings
❏ Parked construction machinery	❏ Frozen ponds, lakes, streams, etc.	
❏ Other: _____		

Would your loved one be attracted to any of these areas?   Yes ____   No ____

Does your neighborhood have sidewalks (or must one walk in the street in order to travel on a hard surface)?

We have sidewalks ____   No sidewalks ____   Both ____

Are there any changes or features in your neighborhood that upset your loved one or for which she has expressed concern?   Yes ____   No ____

❏ New building construction	❏ Loud school events	❏ Neighbor's parties
❏ People walking outside	❏ Children playing outside	❏ Neighbor's yelling
❏ Stray pets seen outside	❏ Landscape or tree trimming crews working	
❏ Children walking home from school	❏ Road construction	
❏ Other _____		

What time of the day do these events or upsets typically occur? _____ AM   _____ PM

What are some of the areas near your home where groups or crowds of people gather?

❏ Shopping center	❏ Subway station	❏ Hotel
❏ School	❏ Military base	❏ Office building
❏ Beach	❏ Public park	❏ Movie theater
❏ Bus stops or depots	❏ Church or temple	❏ Diner or coffee shop
❏ Sport arenas/school event locations	❏ Other (Explain) _____	

Would she attempt to go to such a place or event on her own?   Yes ____   No ____

List things and places that might attract your loved one:

❏ a golf course	❏ children	❏ women	❏ men
❏ pets (dogs, cats, etc.)	❏ a park	❏ a church	❏ a school
❏ stores and malls	❏ a bar	❏ a bench	❏ a bus stop
❏ a former work place	❏ a cemetery	❏ a former home	❏ a beach
❏ wooded areas	❏ a docked boat	❏ a neighborhood shortcut	❏ a farm or field
❏ bodies of water	❏ other _____		

Do you live near a school or other facility which has daily occurrences (such as children arriving or leaving school, buses dropping off children or picking them up, a movie theater which lets out at certain times, etc.)?

Explain _____

_____

What landmarks or neighborhood features would your loved one recognize (e.g., a town square clock, a statue, a fountain, etc.)?

_____

_____

Does or did your loved one ever own property nearby that she inspected or managed? Where is that property?

_____

What is the nearest means of public transportation? How far away is it? _____

❏ Bus stop	❏ Transit train stop	❏ Subway station	❏ Cab
❏ Bus station	❏ Train station	❏ Airport	

❏ Other (Explain) _____

What is the nearest means of your loved one's preferred form of public transportation?

❏ Bus stop	❏ Transit train stop	❏ Subway station	❏ Cab
❏ Bus station	❏ Train station	❏ Airport	

❏ Other (Explain) _____

How far away is it? _____

Would your loved one know how to board or use these forms of transportation?

Yes ____ No ____ How likely is she to attempt it? Very ____ Maybe ____ Unlikely ____

Has she tried to elope taking public transportation in the past?

Yes ____ No ____ When? ____ Where did she want to go? _____

How far did she get? _____

How was she discovered? _____

The Neighborhood *(continued)*

Is there a new or used car dealership nearby?   Yes _____   No _____

Would your loved one be able to convince a dealer to sell her (or let her test drive) a car?

Yes _____   No _____   Unlikely, but possible _____

Dealership	Tel. No.	Address

Is there a car rental office nearby?   Yes _____   No _____

Would your loved one be able to convince a sales person to rent her a car?

Yes _____   No _____   Unlikely, but possible _____

Name	Tel. No.	Address

Take a look outside your home at night *when it is dark.* What areas are illuminated that might attract your loved one at night? Begin by opening each door to the outside and take a look.

Illuminated areas seen from the **front door:**

❑ Street light   ❑ Store light   ❑ Neighbor's house lights

❑ Distant lights   ❑ Other _____

Are these lights kept on all night or do they go off at a certain time? _____

Illuminated areas seen from the **rear door:**

- ❑ Street light   ❑ Store light   ❑ Neighbor's house lights

- ❑ Distant lights   ❑ Other _____

Are these lights kept on all night or do they go off at a certain time? _____

_____

Illuminated areas seen from the **side door:**

- ❑ Street light   ❑ Store light   ❑ Neighbor's house lights

- ❑ Distant lights   ❑ Other _____

Are these lights kept on all night or do they go off at a certain time? _____

_____

Where do the side or rear doors lead? Are there likely directions of travel once one exits from these doors, such as a garage or storage shed or might they lead to a shortcut that leads somewhere else?
Explain _____

_____

_____

What other attractive destinations might be immediately visible from these exits?

_____

_____

_____

_____

NOTES

_____

_____

_____

_____

_____

_____

_____

_____

_____

Family Members   Last Updated: _____

If there is not enough space for all applicable family members, use additional sheets of paper and store them in the workbook.

Spouse or Significant Other

Name _____   Relation _____

Street _____ Unit/Apt. # _____

City _____ State _____ Zip _____

Home Tel. (_____) _____   Cell Phone Number (_____) _____

Bus. Tel. (If applicable)   (_____) _____

Boss/supervisor's name (If applicable) _____

Name loved one uses when referring to spouse/significant other _____

   Alive ____   Deceased ____   If deceased, does LO believe him/her to still be alive? Yes ____   No____

   If deceased, when did he/she die? _____

Does spouse/significant other have any memory or dementia-related issues?

   ❏ Poor memory   ❏ Dementia   ❏ Alzheimer's diagnosis
   ❏ Other _____   ❏ None (no memory or dementia-related issues)

Mother/Father

Name _____   Relation _____

Street _____ Unit/Apt. # _____

City _____ State _____ Zip _____

Home Tel. (_____) _____   Cell Phone Number (_____) _____

Bus. Tel. (_____) _____   Email Address _____

Name loved one uses when referring to this person _____

   Alive ____   Deceased ____   If deceased, does LO believe him/her to still be alive? Yes ____   No____

   If deceased, when did he/she die? _____

Son/Daughter

Name _____ Relation _____

Street _____ Unit/Apt. # _____

City _____ State _____ Zip _____

Home Tel. (_____) _____ Cell Phone Number (_____) _____

Bus. Tel. (_____) _____ Email Address _____

Name loved one uses when referring to this person _____

  Alive _____   Deceased _____   If deceased, does LO believe him/her to still be alive? Yes _____ No_____

  If deceased, when did he/she die? _____

Brother/Sister

Name _____ Relation _____

Street _____ Unit/Apt. # _____

City _____ State _____ Zip _____

Home Tel. (_____) _____ Cell Phone Number (_____) _____

Bus. Tel. (_____) _____ Email Address _____

Name loved one uses when referring to this person _____

  Alive _____   Deceased _____   If deceased, does LO believe him/her to still be alive? Yes _____ No_____

  If deceased, when did he/she die? _____

Brother/Sister

Name _____ Relation _____

Street _____ Unit/Apt. # _____

City _____ State _____ Zip _____

Home Tel. (_____) _____ Cell Phone Number (_____) _____

Bus. Tel. (_____) _____ Email Address _____

Name loved one uses when referring to this person _____

  Alive _____   Deceased _____   If deceased, does LO believe him/her to still be alive? Yes _____ No_____

  If deceased, when did he/she die? _____

Family Members *(continued)*

Aunt/Uncle

Name _____ Relation _____

Street _____ Unit/Apt. # _____

City _____ State _____ Zip _____

Home Tel. (_____) _____ Cell Phone Number (_____) _____

Bus. Tel. (_____) _____ Email Address _____

Name loved one uses when referring to this person _____

   Alive ____   Deceased ____   If deceased, does LO believe him/her to still be alive? Yes ____ No____

   If deceased, when did he/she die? _____

Aunt/Uncle

Name _____ Relation _____

Street _____ Unit/Apt. # _____

City _____ State _____ Zip _____

Home Tel. (_____) _____ Cell Phone Number (_____) _____

Bus. Tel. (_____) _____ Email Address _____

Name loved one uses when referring to this person _____

   Alive ____   Deceased ____   If deceased, does LO believe him/her to still be alive? Yes ____ No____

   If deceased, when did he/she die? _____

Adult Grandchild

Name _____ Relation _____

Street _____ Unit/Apt. # _____

City _____ State _____ Zip _____

Home Tel. (_____) _____ Cell Phone Number (_____) _____

Bus. Tel. (_____) _____ Email Address _____

Name loved one uses when referring to this person _____

   Alive ____   Deceased ____   If deceased, does LO believe him/her to still be alive? Yes ____ No____

   If deceased, when did he/she die? _____

Adult Grandchild

Name _____ Relation _____

Street _____ Unit/Apt. # _____

City _____ State _____ Zip _____

Home Tel. (_____) _____ Cell Phone Number (_____) _____

Bus. Tel. (_____) _____ Email Address _____

Name loved one uses when referring to this person _____

    Alive _____   Deceased _____   If deceased, does LO believe him/her to still be alive? Yes _____ No_____

    If deceased, when did he/she die? _____

Young Grandchildren and Great Grandchildren

Name	Familiar or Nickname	Age

Does your loved one recognize her family members? Yes _____ No _____ Some, but not all _____

    By name? Yes _____ No _____   From photographs? Yes _____ No _____

Does she understand her relationship to these relatives (or does she think her son is her husband, or husband is her father, etc.?) Yes _____ No _____

    Explain _____

_____

_____

    Whom would your loved one most likely seek for comfort and a sense of security?

    Name _____

    Explain _____

_____

_____

Family Members *(continued)*

List the names of family members in the order of LO's ability to recognize them (beginning with the most familiar family member.)

Name	Familiar Name	Relation
1		
2		
3		
4		
5		

NOTES

_____

_____

_____

_____

_____

_____

_____

_____

_____

_____

_____

_____

_____

_____

_____

_____

_____

_____

Part 4

Names and Numbers

Names and Numbers

Last Updated: _____

Who is the designated **Legal Guardian** for your loved one? ❏ None Assigned	Name _____ Tel. No. (_____) _____
Attorney hired to create Legal Guardianship? When was this completed? _____ , _____ Where is document stored? _____ Does Attorney keep a copy? Yes ___ No ___	Name _____ Tel. No. (_____) _____
Who has **Power of Attorney** for your loved one? ❏ None Assigned	Name _____ Tel. No. (_____) _____
Attorney hired to create Power of Attorney? When was this completed? _____ , _____ Where is document stored? _____ Does Attorney keep a copy? Yes ___ No ___	Name _____ Tel. No. (_____) _____

Emergency Contacts

Primary Caregiver—Officials should contact this person FIRST in case of an emergency.

Name		Relation	
Street		Unit/Apt.#	
City	State	Zip	
Home Tel. (_____) _____		Cell Phone Number (_____) _____	
Bus. Tel. (_____) _____		Boss/supervisor's name _____	
		Tel. No. (_____) _____	
Email address		Does this person drive? Yes ___ No ___	

Secondary Contact—If something happened to the primary caregiver, this is the person you would want law enforcement to contact.

Name		Relation	
Street		Unit/Apt.#	
City	State	Zip	
Home Tel. (_____) _____		Cell Phone Number (_____) _____	
Bus. Tel. (_____) _____		Boss/supervisor's name _____	
		Tel. No. (_____) _____	
Email address		Does this person drive? Yes ___ No ___	

Third Contact

Name	Relation
Street	Unit/Apt.#
City	State	Zip

Home Tel. (_____) _____ Cell Phone Number (_____) _____

Bus. Tel. (_____) _____ Boss/supervisor's name _____

Tel. No. (_____) _____

Email address | Does this person drive? Yes _____ No _____

Neighbors' Telephone Numbers—These are the people you might want to call in an emergency to ask if they have seen your loved one (or ask if she is with them).

Name	Address	Tel. No.

Your Friends (people who can be there to support you)

Name	Tel. No.	Cell Phone No.

Community Leaders or Volunteer Search Organizations—who could help law enforcement personnel search for your loved one (consider church or temple groups, Boy/Girl Scout groups, 4-H groups, school clubs, Citizens Observer Patrols—COPS—Neighborhood Watch groups, etc.).

(Team Leader) Name	Group or Club	Tel. No.	Cell Phone No.

Names and Numbers *(continued)*

Support Group Members—If you belong to an Alzheimer's Support Group, here is a group of people who share your concern, know exactly what you are going through, and would be very quick to help you (as you would be to help them if the situation were reversed).

Name	Tel. No.	Cell Phone No.

Other Important People (Miscellaneous Numbers)

Description	Name	Tel. No.	Cell Phone No.
Housekeeper/Cleaning Person			
Yard Man			
Doorman/woman			
Family Doctor			
Geriatrician			
Other Doctor _____			
Other Doctor _____			
Family Attorney			
Elderlaw Attorney			
Local Alzheimer's Org.			
Area Agency on Aging			
Geriatric Care Manager			
Police or Sheriff's Dept. (Non-Emergency No.)			
Building Manager			
Building Superintendent			
Bldg. Maintenance Dept.			

For those living in gated communities

Description	Name	Tel. No.
Gatehouse Personnel		
Security Department		
Maintenance Department		
Manager		

Hired Caregivers

1. Name _____ Tel. No. (____) _____

Street _____ Cell No. (____) _____

City _____ State ____ Zip ____ Hours _____ to _____

Days of the week: Mon. ___ Tues. ___ Wed. ___ Thurs. ___ Fri. ___ Sat. ___ Sun. ___

How long has this person worked for you? _____ Does your loved one like this caregiver? Yes ___ No ___

Is there a familiar name that LO uses to refer to this person? _____

2. Name _____ Tel. No. (____) _____

Street _____ Cell No. (____) _____

City _____ State ____ Zip ____ Hours _____ to _____

Days of the week: Mon. ___ Tues. ___ Wed. ___ Thurs. ___ Fri. ___ Sat. ___ Sun. ___

How long has this person worked for you? _____ Does your loved one like this caregiver? Yes ___ No ___

Is there a familiar name that LO uses to refer to this person? _____

NOTES

Names and Numbers *(continued)*

Day Care

Does your loved one attend daycare? Yes _____ No _____

Name of daycare center _____

Street _____ Apt. # _____

City _____ State _____ Zip _____

Tel. No. (_____) _____ Hours _____ to _____

Days of the week: Mon. _____ Tues. _____ Wed. _____ Thurs. _____ Fri. _____ Sat. _____ Sun. _____

Emergency or after hours telephone number: (_____) _____

What term do you use when referring to the daycare center?

("We are going to the _____")

What term does your loved one use when referring to the daycare center (e.g., "work," "the office," "school,"

etc.)? _____

Does your loved one like going to the daycare center?   Yes _____ No _____

Is your loved one picked up by a driver? Yes _____ No _____   Name: _____

What time is your loved one typically picked up? _____

What time is your loved one typically dropped off at home? _____

Hospitals (provide information for local hospitals)

Name	Gen. Tel. No.	Emergency Room Tel. No.

NOTES

_____

_____

_____

_____

Consider places within your community where a Good Samaritan might take a confused, elderly person who was found wandering or lost, including:

❏ nursing homes

❏ homeless shelters

❏ churches & temples

❏ fire station

❏ seniors centers

❏ senior daycare centers

❏ police station

❏ mental facilities

❏ hospitals

❏ Area Agency on Aging offices

❏ Alzheimer's Assn. office

❏ Other Alz. org. offices

Name	Address	Tel. No.

Telephone numbers of **Local Cab, Bus and Transit Companies**—to notify (to be on the lookout) or ask if any of their drivers saw or picked up your loved one.

Type of Company	Name	Telephone Number
Cab		
Cab		
Bus		
Bus		
Airport limo service		
Other*		

* Non-emergency transportation companies, such as Good Wheels, Transportation for People with Disabilities, Dial-A-Ride, and transportation companies for the elderly.

People Your Loved One Might Seek   Last Updated: _____

Which family member might your loved one turn to or seek for help, if he could not find you?

_____

Whom might your loved one seek or approach for help (other than the primary caregiver)?

❏ clergy   ❏ a friend   ❏ spouse   ❏ a family member

❏ doctor   ❏ a neighbor   ❏ a uniformed professional   ❏ maid or hired help

❏ anyone   ❏ other: _____

When frightened, whom would your loved one request? _____

What name would he use to refer to this person? _____

Who would you say is your loved one's **best friend**? _____

(Provide information on this person, if not already provided. Use an extra sheet of paper.)

_____

_____

Is there anyone in your loved one's life (other than spouse) that he is romantically attracted to or has expressed a romantic interest in lately? Yes _____ No _____

Explain: _____

_____

Friends (include information on important friends of your loved one—from the past, as well—especially if their names have been recently mentioned)

Name _____

Street _____ Unit/Apt. # _____

City _____ State _____ Zip _____

Home Tel. (_____) _____ Cell Phone Number (_____) _____

Bus. Tel.   (_____) _____ E-mail address _____

Alive _____   Deceased _____   If deceased, does LO believe this person to still be alive? Yes _____ No _____

If deceased, when did he/she die? _____

Name loved one uses when referring to this person _____

How far away does/did this person live from loved one? _____ blocks _____ miles

Does loved one visit or speak of visiting this person? Yes _____ No _____

Has loved one traveled to this person's house or apartment within the last few years? Yes _____ No _____

How long ago? _____

Friends *(continued)*

Name _____

Street _____ Unit/Apt. # _____

City _____ State _____ Zip _____

Home Tel. (_____) _____ Cell Phone Number (_____) _____

Bus. Tel. (_____) _____ E-mail address _____

Alive _____ Deceased _____ If deceased, does LO believe this person to still be alive? Yes _____ No _____

If deceased, when did he/she die? _____

Name loved one uses when referring to this person _____

How far away does/did this person live from loved one? _____ blocks _____ miles

Does loved one visit or speak of visiting this person? Yes _____ No _____

Has loved one traveled to this person's house or apartment within the last few years? Yes _____ No _____

How long ago? _____

Other People Your Loved One May Seek

Name _____

Street _____ Unit/Apt. # _____

City _____ State _____ Zip _____

Home Tel. (_____) _____ Cell Phone Number (_____) _____

Bus. Tel. (_____) _____ E-mail address _____

Alive _____ Deceased _____ If deceased, does LO believe this person to still be alive? Yes _____ No _____

If deceased, when did he/she die? _____

Name loved one uses when referring to this person _____

How far away does/did this person live from loved one? _____ blocks _____ miles

Does loved one visit or speak of visiting this person? Yes _____ No _____

Has loved one traveled to this person's house or apartment within the last few years? Yes _____ No _____

How long ago? _____

People Your Loved One Might Seek *(continued)*

List (in order) the people you think your loved one might attempt or want to go visit. (If their information is not already provided, please use an extra sheet of paper or space at the end of this section to add it.)

	Name	Familiar Name	Telephone Number
1			
2			
3			
4			
5			
6			
7			
8			

NOTES

Interacting With Your Loved One

Interacting with Your Loved One

Last Updated: _____

The following questions and information are designed to help community or law enforcement personnel understand limitations **to communicating with your loved one once he is found and actions that could potentially upset him.**

Communication

What are your recommendations for communicating with your loved one:

❏ Ask only "yes" or "no" questions   ❏ Repeat information   ❏ Be very patient

❏ Use gestures and body language   ❏ Use short sentences   ❏ Speak slowly

❏ Use simple and familiar words   ❏ Speak in a soft, calm, reassuring voice

❏ Stand in front of loved one when   ❏ Identify yourself frequently (by name
   speaking to him   and who you are)

❏ Refer to him by his title (e.g., "Judge Adams," "Mr. Smith")   ❏ Use his first name

❏ Can your loved one provide reliable answers to simple questions?   Yes ____   No ____

❏ Loved one tends to always answer "No" or "Yes" (Which one? "Yes" ____ or "No" ____)

Would your loved one respond better to a male ____ or female ____?

Does your loved one understand English?   Yes ____   No ____

What is the primary language of your loved one? _____

What is the current language of choice for your loved one?_____

What languages other than English does your loved one speak? _____

Has there been a recent increase in the use of this language? Yes ____   No ____

Difficulties and Challenges (Identify tasks and functions which are troublesome for your loved one):

❏ expressing fears or concerns   ❏ speaking intelligibly

❏ understanding spoken sentences   ❏ paying attention/staying focused

❏ understanding people who talk fast   ❏ understanding people with accents

❏ performing simple tasks   ❏ standing for extended periods

❏ comprehending too much information   ❏ remembering information

❏ understanding long sentences   ❏ standing up (from seated position)

❏ following a train of thought   ❏ making choices (from more than two options)

❏ toileting   ❏ eating

❏ walking   ❏ sitting down

❏ following instructions   ❏ reading

❏ explaining things   ❏ balance

❏ remaining seated   ❏ expressing concerns

❏ dressing   ❏ other _____

Bothersome Factors (Identify things or events that may upset or frighten your loved one)

❏ loud noises	❏ aggressive behavior	❏ shouting
❏ traffic	❏ strangers	❏ having his hand/arm held
❏ crowds	❏ being corrected	❏ too many questions
❏ bright lights	❏ background noise	❏ glare
❏ animals (dogs, horses)	❏ car headlights	❏ sudden movements
❏ flashing lights/sirens	❏ radio "chatter"	❏ people crying
❏ darkness	❏ children	❏ standing for too long
❏ people in uniform	❏ his reflection in a mirror	❏ being handcuffed

❏ people of different ethnicity _____

❏ other _____

Does your loved one suffer from Sundowning or Sundown Syndrome?   Yes ____   No ____

Has your loved one ever been arrested or in trouble with the law?   Yes ____   No ____

Does he harbor any anger or hostility towards police officers?   Yes ____   No ____

How might your loved one act out if he were upset?

❏ hitting	❏ name calling	❏ verbal abuse/cursing	❏ spitting
❏ grabbing	❏ attempt to get up & leave	❏ yelling for help	❏ crying
❏ fleeing	❏ silence (clamming up)	❏ kicking	❏ moaning
❏ screaming	❏ throwing objects	❏ other _____	

How capable is your loved one of outwitting casual supervision?   Likely ____   Unlikely ____

Is your loved one likely to try to escape from rescue personnel?   Yes ____   No ____

What tends to calm or pacify your loved one when he is upset?

❏ newspaper	❏ children	❏ pets	❏ magazine	❏ humor
❏ doll	❏ music	❏ television	❏ radio	❏ looking at pictures

❏ food (what kind of food?—ice cream, for example) _____

❏ candy (favorite candy or candy bar) _____

❏ other (explain) _____

What are your loved one's favorite topics of conversation? (spouse, son, daughter, hobbies, career, hometown)
(Include names) _____

_____

Are there topics of conversation that should be avoided (that upset your loved one)? Explain.

_____

_____

*"My advice to people who are caregivers is that . . .
really . . . just keep things under control. Keep things
easy to understand—not baby language or something
like that. Don't talk down to us. Don't get mad when
we forget things—because getting mad is part of
Alzheimer's."*[1]

Cary Smith Henderson
Author and Alzheimer's disease sufferer

Tips for Enhancing Communication

One thing to realize and understand is that people with Alzheimer's disease are not crazy or stupid—they have a disease of the brain and as such may be easily overwhelmed or confused. So just as you would not overcompensate for someone with another disability, do not overcompensate for the person with dementia—she *will* notice it and react. Among the abilities that people with Alzheimer's retain long into the disease is the keen ability to recognize and respond to body language—both good and bad.

People with Alzheimer's disease often find it difficult to express themselves and understand others. They may:

- Have difficulty finding the right words
- Use familiar words repeatedly
- Invent new words to describe familiar objects
- Frequently lose their train of thought
- Experience difficulty organizing words logically
- Make racially, sexually, or otherwise inappropriate comments
- Revert to speaking in a native language
- Curse or use offensive words
- Speak less often
- Rely on nonverbal gestures

Suggestions:

- Keep things simple.
- Use short sentences and familiar words.
- Break tasks and instructions into clear, simple steps.
- Ask one question at a time.
- Show that you are listening and trying to understand what is being said.
- Be careful not to interrupt.

---

1. Cary Smith Henderson, *Partial View: An Alzheimer's Journal,* Dallas, TX: Southern Methodist University Press, 1998, p. 86.

- Allow enough time for a response.
- Encourage the person to continue to express thoughts even if she is having difficulty.
- Avoid criticizing, correcting, or arguing.
- Be calm and supportive.
- Use a gentle, relaxed tone of voice.
- Use positive, friendly facial expressions.
- Always approach the person from the front.
- Identify yourself, insert periodic reminders of your name.
- Address her by name.
- Speak warmly, slowly, and clearly.
- Maintain eye contact.
- Avoid using pronouns—identify people by their names (including relations—such as "your son, John").
- Avoid using negative statements and quizzing (e.g., "You know who that is, don't you?").
- Use nonverbal communication such as pointing.
- Offer assistance only as needed.
- Don't talk about the person as if she isn't there.
- Be patient, flexible and understanding.
- If accepted, use a gentle, reassuring hand or shoulder touch.
- Understand that it is all right to go or play along with whatever the patient is thinking or saying, whether based on reality or not.

NOTES

_____

_____

_____

_____

_____

_____

_____

_____

_____

_____

_____

_____

_____

NOTES

Part 6

Searching for a
Lost Loved One

Searching for a Lost Loved One

The search for a missing Alzheimer's patient is not a typical missing person search. Not only is the person likely to be frightened and confused, but he is not missing by his own choice.

There are different levels of searches for a missing Alzheimer's patient, as well as a myriad of tools, equipment and strategies available to the experts, including different types of scent dogs, helicopters, infrared heat detectors, etc. Once a loved one is discovered missing it is advisable and well worth calling in the pros.

Levels of Searches

1.   What can you do?
2.   What can law enforcement and fire/rescue do?
3.   What can search & rescue do?

Level One: What You Can Do

You can take *immediate* steps to search your home and yard. You can also call neighbors, friends and family—asking if they have seen your loved one and if they can help you find him. Ask them to get into their cars and conduct a visual patrol of the area. Make sure that they have your telephone and cell phone number, in case they find your loved one.

Most missing Alzheimer's patients (on foot) are found within one mile of their home (or point last seen). The sooner you notify authorities, the less distance your lived one can travel (minimizing the area needed to be searched) and maximizing the likelihood of his quick and safe discovery.

Do not try to organize and execute your own search—leave this up to the experts. Call 911 and get law enforcement involved as soon as possible.

Level Two: Law Enforcement and Fire/Rescue

It's important to understand that some law enforcement and fire/rescue jurisdictions may only be able to look out for (not search for) a missing loved one—to the limits that their resources and availability of personnel will allow. Though not the case for all police and sheriff's departments, this may mean that only available officers can patrol limited areas, knock on some doors and "Be On the Lookout" (BOLO) for your loved one. They may or may not have the personnel or resources to perform a complete, organized search.

Also, it is important to realize that law enforcement and fire/rescue may be different entities from search and rescue teams—each with their own expertises, limitations, and specialized resources.

That said, one of the most important steps to finding a missing loved one with Alzheimer's is to call the police or sheriff's department as soon as possible—no more than 15 minutes from the time your loved one is discovered missing.

Level Three: Search & Rescue (SAR)

Search and rescue teams called in to search for your loved one can perform a complete, organized search. These are specialized teams whose expertise is to design and execute a search for a missing individual. Their resources include "trackers," teams of people and dogs, and proven tactics to carefully and systematically cover defined areas. SAR teams will map the area into grids, identify likely destinations, interview neighbors and friends, determine direction of travel, calculate the rate of travel, and discover clues, and in many cases, they will best understand and be able to interpret the clues and information that you provide in this workbook.

If it is necessary to use specialized SAR teams to find your loved one, the sooner they can be brought in, the more likely it will be that they will find him and bring him home safe and sound.

The responsibility and decision to call in specialized search and rescue teams falls upon your local law enforcement. Once they determine that an "endangered missing person" cannot be found, only they can authorize the use of specialized SAR teams.

Steps to Take When Your Loved One Is Discovered Missing

Immediate Steps:

- If you (or a neighbor) have a swimming pool, check it immediately, as well as other areas of imminent danger, such as the bottom of stairs, etc.

- From your front yard, look up and down your street.

- Check to see if any vehicles are missing.

- Do an initial but thorough search of your home. Check every room, including rooms that are not often used, such as laundry or utility rooms and closets. Check all potential hiding places, such as under the bed (your loved one may be hiding from you, as well).

- Open and search all locked rooms within your home. It may have been your loved one (on the other side) who locked the door.

- In condominium or multi-story buildings, be sure to check all unlocked doors, including those to community storage rooms, utility rooms, electric rooms, doors leading to stairwells and building exits, which may open freely from the inside, but are locked from the outside.

- Call or check your next-door neighbors to see if your loved one happened to walk into the wrong house, apartment or condominium by mistake. Leave your telephone number in case they think of something new or they see your loved one.

- If you live in a gated community call the security department and gate house personnel to inquire if they have seen your loved one.

- Check outside:

○ sheds	○ barns	○ storm shelters
○ staircases	○ trailers	○ secluded or heavily landscaped
○ garage	○ cellars	areas of your yard
○ stairwells	○ attics	
○ basements	○ parked cars	

- Write down the time your loved one was discovered missing.

TIP:
Always carry your cell phone with you.

After 15 Minutes:

- Dial 911 to notify law enforcement and fire rescue. Do not wait. The longer you wait, the further away your loved one can travel.

- If you have a cell phone, give the police or sheriff's department that number as well as your home number.

- Stay at home and wait for law enforcement personnel to arrive for the initial interview.

- Call a friend or family member to be with you, support you, and provide assistance. This is no time for you to be acting alone.

- When law enforcement officials arrive, show them your completed workbook.

- Notify families in your building and neighborhood. Ask them if they have seen your loved one or if she is at their house (especially if you live in a development or community where the homes or apartments all look similar).

- Ask friends/family members to patrol the roads (by car) within a three-block radius (in urban areas) and a one-half-mile radius (in rural areas). Observe yards and areas on each side of the road carefully. Check the locations identified as Immediate Neighborhood Dangers (and the routes to them) on page 56.

- Create a list of the names *and cell phone numbers* of all key personnel, friends, and family members who are helping in the search to find your loved one. This list will come in very handy once your loved one is found and you have to notify everyone of the good news. (Use the forms on page 67 or create one of your own.)

- Provide neighbors, gatehouse and security personnel in your development/building with photos of your loved one. Include your telephone and cell phone number and ask them to call you if they see your loved one.

- Assign friends/family members to ask the postman/woman, workers, delivery drivers, children playing, and others in the neighborhood if they have seen your loved one walking by himself (bring a photo to show them). Neighborhood children can be valuable eyes and ears (they also know the best places in the neighborhood to hide and can check them out, often in less time than the law enforcement or search & rescue personnel).

- Have a friend or family member call cab companies and local stores/restaurants that have delivery services to instruct their drivers to be on the lookout for your loved one.

Make sure that there is always someone remaining at your home to receive phone calls, answer questions or notify family and searchers in case your loved one suddenly returns home or is found.

- Check routes to previous residences, work locations and places frequently visited or mentioned by your loved one. Also consider routes that your loved one believes would lead him to "home" or these locations.

- Call Safe Return (whether your loved one is registered with them or not) at (800) 572-1122 to report that your loved one with AD is missing. This information will be entered into a national database which could help find him in the event that he crosses state lines. Also provide Safe Return with the names of law enforcement and lead rescue personnel involved in the search. (If your loved one is registered with a local Alzheimer's organization wanderer ID program, call them as well.)

- Call your local Alzheimer's organization, Alzheimer's Association local chapter or Alzheimer's resource center to notify them of your loved one's disappearance. Consider asking them to send a staff member to be with you and to help you during this time of need.

- Limit your use of the telephone to only important calls in order to keep the line open.

- If you live in a building or development with multiple families, place flyers in key locations.

- Do not straighten or clean up your loved one's bedroom. Check the room carefully to look for your loved one, but leave the room and bed as is. Do not change or launder the sheets, bedding or night clothing.

After 1 Hour:

- Call neighbors, community leaders and contact numbers listed in this workbook to provide additional support (for you and your family) and assistance to law enforcement.

- Ask the police or sheriff's department if they have an Emergency Notification System or "Communicator"—a high speed phone-dialing system that can be programmed to call homes and businesses in a specific area and deliver a pre-recorded emergency message alerting them of your loved one's disappearance. (Refer to the information on A Child Is Missing Program on page 135.)

- Expand the (family and friends) vehicle search to include the area within a one-mile radius (and then two miles) from the point last seen. (The average distance a person can travel in an hour is two miles.) Begin at the outside and work your way in towards the point last seen. Don't become lax in re-searching the original areas when expanding the search.

- For searches taking place in urban areas, ask the police or sheriff's department if they have checked and notified local hospitals, bus and taxi companies.

- Ask and give permission to the police or sheriff's department PIO (Press Information Officer) to contact your local media (TV, radio and newspapers).

- Ask law enforcement if there is an Amber Alert system in your community that can be used to send a message to news agencies, highway signs and television stations to notify the entire community to be on the lookout for your missing loved one.

- Ask the police or sheriff's department if they have checked local jails or holding cells, just to make sure that your loved one was not detained (perhaps because he was unable to give his name and was thought to be intoxicated).

- Ask the law enforcement team if they have requested specialized search and rescue personnel to become involved yet. If your loved one has not been found within one hour, perhaps it is time to consider going to the next step.

After 24 Hours:

- Print and put up flyers in your community and in the windows of local stores (refer to the sample of a missing persons flyer on page 115).

- Ask a friend or family member to *again* patrol the area by car within a one-mile radius of the point your loved one was last seen. (Remember: Most lost Alzheimer's wanderers are found within one mile of the point last seen.)

- If search dogs are being used, provide an item of your loved one's *worn and unlaundered* clothing (a shirt, blouse, T-shirt, socks, underwear or pillowcase). *Do not handle it yourself,* just lead the search team to it.

Do not organize your own searches.
Let the professionals do what they do best.

- After two days you should notify your county medical examiner or coroner *in writing.* This has two purposes—to notify law enforcement officials and to inform you in the event that the descriptions of your loved one do or do not match any of their unidentified deceased victims. An example of such a letter can be found on page 121.

Once Your Loved One Is Found

- Notify Safe Return and all other organizations involved in the search.

- If you have involved community volunteers, notify them that your loved one has been found. (Call the cell phone numbers collected at the beginning of the search.)

- If your loved one is found by someone other than law enforcement personnel, be sure to notify law enforcement immediately.

- Once your loved one is found, you may be asked to come pick him up. If so, you should remember to bring along certain items, including:

○ a fresh adult brief	○ shoes or slippers	○ a clean change of clothing
○ a warm coat or jacket	○ a blanket	○ a candy bar or snack

  ○ medications (if there is an urgency for your loved one to take them)
  ○ appropriate food if meds need to be ground up and taken with food to be swallowed
  ○ your loved one's wheelchair, walker or cane
  ○ his favorite _____ (whatever that may be)
  ○ If he needs to be hospitalized, bring insurance and medical information.

- When reunited with your loved one:
  ○ Do not scold him;
  ○ Do not become overly emotional or tell him how worried you were (to avoid further upsetting him);
  ○ Make him comfortable (provide a snack, change his clothes and briefs, if necessary);
  ○ Provide any necessary medications;
  ○ Calmly take him home;
  ○ Reassure him that everything is all right;
  ○ If possible, identify the cause or trigger for the elopement.

- Remove or ask a friend or family member to remove flyers that were posted in the community.

- Take steps to prevent and alert the caregiver of attempts to wander away from home in the future (see the section on Preparing and Planning Ahead—pages 99–103).

- If your loved one does not want to go home, go for a short stroll or drive, stop for ice cream, or head "somewhere else" and stop at home on the way.

> **Once a person with Alzheimer's leaves home and is unable or unwilling to return, or becomes lost,**
> **it is likely that it will happen again.**
> **Take the necessary precautions.**

Additional Search Tips

There are no set rules that apply to the wandering patterns of people with Alzheimer's disease, but there are hypotheses and observations that have been helpful in past searches. Here are a few suggestions:

- If you live in a residential building where all the doors look alike, ask a friend or family member to check to see if your loved one is in someone else's apartment, condo, etc. (Check nearby units and units in the same location on different floors.)

- Do not underestimate your loved one's ability or intent to hide. And remember that he may not respond to someone calling out his name.

- Check dense foliage and heavily wooded areas. Some lost wanderers have been found in areas so thick with briar bushes and overgrowth that even search dogs refused to go into them. Do not overlook these areas, particularly those close to and adjacent to roads or paths.

- Check behind bushes, low walls, and areas adjacent to roads. Often people with AD are found short distances from roads (within 30 feet).

- Check the bottom of areas that slope down from roads and pathways. Sometimes people with Alzheimer's will lose their balance and wind up at the bottom of a ditch, hill, or slope. (The incline does not have to be very much to cause a loss of balance.)

- Pay particular attention to physical features that can be followed, including roads, paths, low walls, fences, and railroad tracks.

- Pay particular attention to locations where paths come to an end (or dead-end) or run into an obstacle that would have to be walked around or climbed or would otherwise cause someone to stop or make a decision. People with AD tend to continue going in one general direction or follow a path, until they run into an obstacle. At that time they often stop right where they are or hide close by.

- Check makeshift shelters, including storage and tool sheds, parked cars, bus stops, pay phone booths, ATM lobbies, and parking lots (between and even in cars).

- Check local restaurants, diners, convenience stores, and places that your loved one frequents or may have gone on an errand.

- Call local hospitals, nursing homes, shelters and other places where a Good Samaritan might take an elderly person if they found him lost.

- Open spaces are alluring. People with AD tend to follow paths of least resistance and avoid obstacles. Be particularly alert to open areas, such as fields, parks, drainage ditches, streams, creek beds, etc.

- People with AD will often head for "familiar" destinations. Pay special attention to "favorite" (not necessarily the correct or most direct) routes and short-cuts to places where your loved one may want to go.

- Checked "perceived" destinations—It may not be the actual route to a destination that is important, but rather your loved one's *perceived* route that *he* thinks will lead him to "home," work, school, etc.

- Some experts report that traveling downhill is more common than uphill, hypothesizing that it is easier.

- What exit door did your loved one most likely use when leaving? By providing an initial clue to his direction, you can increase the odds of finding your loved one (however, do not rely on this 100%—he could always have left through another door).

- Calling out your loved one's name may not be effective. He may hide from people trying to find him, feel that if caught he will get in trouble, not be able to hear you or simply not recognize his own name (or the people looking for him).

> **Don't take anything for granted.**
> In a Florida study, out of 675 missing Alzheimer's wanderers,
> approximately 26% were found in a neighbor's yard; 22% were
> found walking on the street; 12% at businesses; and 9% in a hospital
> or healthcare facility. Eighty percent walked away, 10% used
> public transportation, and 5% got into cars and drove away.[1]

Survival Factors

The most important criteria contributing to the safe return of your loved one include:

- Elapsed Time—The longer you wait or that it takes to notify law enforcement that your loved one is missing, the farther away your loved one can travel.

- Weather Conditions—Most missing persons with Alzheimer's who do not survive die from hypothermia (in cold weather), hyperthermia (in warm weather), exhaustion or dehydration.

- Co-existing Medical Conditions—Alzheimer's is an age-related disease. Therefore, if a person is old enough to have one age-related condition, he is old enough to have another—which may affect his ability to survive on his own.

---

1. Meredeth A. Rowe, RN, PhD, Judith C. Glover, RN, MS, "Antecedents, descriptions and consequences of wandering in cognitively-impaired adults and the Safe Return Program," *American Journal of Alzheimer's Disease and Other Dementias,* Vol. 16, No. 6, November/December, 2001.

- Environmental Dangers—Swimming pools, traffic, dense woods, cliffs, bodies of water, creek beds, and drainage ditches, etc. are all dangers and/or obstacles to finding a missing person. If in close proximity to the point last seen, such areas should be searched immediately.

> Fishing and boat docks pose a unique danger in that they represent a path with only a deadly end. The person with Alzheimer's may unknowingly continue walking, right off the end of the dock, not realizing that it comes to a stop.

- Regional Dangers—Certain regions of the country have unique dangers, including:

    Predatory animals (bears in wooded areas, mountain lions in mountainous regions, and even alligators in southern Florida).

    Farmlands might include cattle fields or pens where your loved one might be trampled by horses, cows or even hogs.

    Rural areas might present places that are not in themselves dangerous, but make it more difficult to find someone, such as vast corn or wheat fields, swamp lands or dense woods.

- Age vs. Stage of AD—Surprisingly, the older person's age is not a strong indicator of the distance that he may travel. However, the stage of Alzheimer's that he is in may be. People in the middle and later stages of Alzheimer's tend to travel shorter distances.

- Trackable Wander-Alerting Devices—If your loved one is wearing a trackable wander-alerting device, this will substantially increase the speed and the searchers' ability to find him (see pages 102 and 142).

- Identification and Wandering Jewelry—Enrollment in the Safe Return program provides an ID bracelet or necklace with an 800 number and customer ID, which can be valuable if your loved one is discovered by law enforcement personnel or a Good Samaritan. (See pages 124–125 for more information on Wanderer ID bracelet programs.)

NOTES

_____

_____

_____

_____

_____

_____

_____

_____

_____

NOTES

Part 7

Helping a Lost Wanderer

Helping a Lost Wanderer

People with Alzheimer's disease wandering in public will likely be confused or frightened or may have impaired ability to communicate. If they are approached in a manner that they perceive as threatening, they may try to escape or become combative.

People with Alzheimer's disease *are not crazy or stupid*. Alzheimer's is not a mental illness, it is a neurological disease (a disease of the brain) which makes it difficult for those with the disease to understand and process information.

When encountering a person with Alzheimer's who appears lost or confused:

- Assess the situation. (Does the person need help?)

- Check to see if she is wearing an Alzheimer's bracelet.

- Ask her if there is someone that you can call for her.

- If allowed, check for clothing name/telephone labels or ask if she has an ID card in her purse or wallet.

- If it is determined that the person needs help, call 911.

- Stay with the person until help arrives—be a friend to her.

- Treat her with *respect* and *concern*—offer to help.

- Speak slowly and clearly.

- Act in a calm and reassuring manner. She will be cued by the tone of your voice and body language.

- Approach her from the front to avoid startling her.

- Act as if you know her—if you know her name, use it ("Hi, Mary. How are you?").

- State the reason for your encounter ("You look like you could use some help. Can I help you?"— or ask her to help you).

- Identify yourself—tell her or remind her of your name (perhaps more than once).

- Ask one question at a time, preferably simple "yes" or "no" questions.

- If necessary, repeat the question.

- Avoid asking too many questions.

- Make suggestions ("Let's go over here where we can sit down," etc).
  If her conversation makes no sense, *just go with it* (do not try to correct her):

  > *Person with AD:* "Those people want to hurt me."
  > *You:* "Oh my, let's go over here where it's safe."

- Move the person away from traffic, crowds, and noisy environments.

- Look for identification: an ID bracelet, nursing home or hospital wristband, ID card, or personalized clothing labels. If she is wearing a Safe Return bracelet, check the back. It will have the person's first name, ID number and emergency toll-free number.

- Don't take the person's word that she is all right. People with Alzheimer's can:

  be injured, but unable to communicate their condition,

  forget that they had an accident, despite the injury,

  be unable to make the association between discomfort and the injury causing it.

- Dial 911 and notify the police or sheriff's department. They may already be looking for this person and can help return her safely home.

And finally, understand that if the person is trying to escape from a perceived danger/threat or determined to go to a specific destination, going home may not be something that she wants or is willing to do.

NOTES

_____

_____

_____

_____

_____

_____

_____

_____

_____

_____

_____

_____

_____

_____

_____

_____

_____

_____

_____

_____

_____

_____

NOTES

Part 8

Preparing and Planning Ahead

Preparing and Planning Ahead

Have a Plan

What would you do if one morning or one evening you discovered that your loved one was missing—nowhere to be found?

- What steps would you take?
- Whom would you call?
- What would be the first and most important things to do?

Now is the time to think about this and to create a plan, not when it happens, in the heat of the dilemma. Perhaps this workbook can offer some guidance, good ideas, and suggestions.

Listen to Your Loved One—Alzheimer's is a disease that changes people. Though you may know the person that you lived with or were married to for the last 10, 20, 30 or more years, within the last few days things may have changed. He may have new concerns, fears, needs, desires, etc. Often the clues and red flags are there, we just don't hear them.

Be Prepared

Should the need ever occur, you should be prepared to instantly search your home and surrounding area—rain or shine, day or night. The bottom line is that you need to be prepared in case you have to dash outside quickly to find or catch your fleeing loved one. You can't afford to waste time looking for your shoes or coat. Every second counts.

- Among the most important tools for a nighttime search is a flashlight. Have one ready, stocked with fresh batteries, stored in a location where it can be quickly and easily found. (We recommend a 3- or 4-battery Mag-Lite flashlight—available at your home improvement center. They are durable and provide a high-intensity beam.)

- For inclement weather, keep the season-appropriate apparel convenient. These might include boots, a warm coat, an umbrella, etc.

- Notify security, gate house personnel, neighbors and neighborhood children who typically play outside to let you know if they ever see your loved one out walking by himself. (Do this periodically, in case personnel change and as a reminder.)

- If you live in a building or community where homes or doors look alike, make yours unique:
    1. Place a visible plaque next to the door with your loved one's name on it (e.g., "John's House").
    2. Put something bright and colorful next to the door or in front of the house.
    3. Every time that you go outside with your loved one, make a comment and point these features out to him.

- Use "neighborhood alerts"—ask neighbors, delivery personnel, children who play outside, gate-house/security employees and your mail carrier to let you know if they ever see your loved one roaming in the neighborhood.

- Visit your doctor and fill out a Medical Release Form (see pages 119–120) for your loved one. Ask your doctor to keep it on file. This can save a lot of time and trouble in the event that law enforcement needs a copy of your loved one's medical information.

- Purchase a trackable wandering alarm (see pages 102 and 142).

- Enroll in the Safe Return Program (see pages 124–125) or your local Alzheimer's organization Wander ID program.

- Attach pieces of iron-on reflective tape to the back and front of your loved one's favorite jacket, cap, shoes, etc. Use adhesive-backed reflective tape for his wheelchair, walker, and cane. To purchase reflective tape:

  > Check your local bicycle supply store; or
  > Go to www.identi-tape.com or call (877) 964-8273; or
  > Go to www.ghsports.com or call (877) 428-9447; or
  > Go to www.reflectivelyyours.com or call (518) 399-9339.

- Purchase a "special" fluorescent-colored cap for you and your loved one to wear when going out in public. Such a bright, easy-to-see hat will make it easier to spot him if you unexpectedly become separated. (Buying one for yourself to wear also might make it more acceptable for him to wear this "crazy" cap.)

- Keep a few pairs of worn, unwashed articles of clothing in a sealed plastic bag, in case they are needed for scent dogs. These might include a shirt, blouse, T-shirt, socks, underwear or a pillowcase. Facilities should keep such an article in a separate bag for each resident.

- Have duplicate keys made to any and all lockable rooms, sheds, storm shelters, etc., where your loved one might lock himself in. Store them in a safe place and label each one.

- If you have a cell phone, purchase an extra battery and keep it charged.

- Provide neighbors, gatehouse, and security personnel in your development with photos of your loved one. Include your phone number and a note asking them to call you if he is seen walking by himself:

  "If you see this man walking by himself, call _____ immediately."[1]

- Fill out your workbook and keep it updated.

Take Photos—Take pictures of your loved one. Make several copies and keep them in this workbook. If ever needed, they can be given to or shown to law enforcement personnel, neighborhood children, and people in your community. Put an address sticker on the back of each photo with your name, telephone number, and cell phone number.

Create a video of your loved one and store it in a convenient location. It can be used by television stations that broadcast alerts.

Credit Cards—Use a copy machine to make a copy of your loved one's credit cards. Keep it in this workbook. These can be checked by law enforcement officials to see if and where there is any credit card activity after your loved one is discovered missing. (Black out the expiration date to ensure that the credit card numbers cannot be used by anyone with access to this information.)

---

1. M.L. Warner, *The Complete Guide to Alzheimer's-Proofing Your Home.* Purdue University Press, 2000, p. 248.

ID's, Address Labels and Name Tags

- Put ID cards in your loved one's jacket (pocket), wallet or purse, complete with his current address, an emergency telephone number and your cell phone number.

- Order address labels *with your telephone number and cell phone number.* There are many companies that offer them at very reasonable prices. (A number of charitable organizations offer free address labels, including the United Spinal Association, Paralyzed Veterans of America and the American Diabetes Association.)

- Place these address labels on your loved one's walker, wheelchair, cane, cell phone and anything else that he may carry with him.

- Sew or iron on name tags in items of clothing, purses, hats, scarves, each shoe, etc. (The Safe Return Program provides iron-on clothing labels.)

- Whenever going out into public with your loved one make sure that she is wearing and carrying identification:

  a Safe Return bracelet *and*

  clothing labels *and*

  an identification card in her purse or wallet.

NOTES

_____

_____

_____

_____

_____

_____

_____

_____

_____

_____

_____

_____

_____

_____

_____

_____

Preventing Future Episodes of Elopement

Once a person with Alzheimer's is identified as being prone or likely to wander away from her home or caregiver, it is important that steps be taken to ensure that it never happens again.

- Stay close to your loved one when taking her to the mall, stores, public events, etc. Remember, it just takes a split second to disappear and get lost in a crowd or turn a corner.

- When you do take your loved one out, dress her in a bright, colorful, easy-to-see cap and clothing to help you find her just in case you become separated.

- Pay close attention to your loved one when she becomes agitated. This is a time when she is more likely to walk out of the house (in anger). If she does go outside, go after her immediately. Do not ever assume that you know where she is going or that she will return shortly.

- If there is any chance that your loved one might try to drive off in the family car:

  Install a "secret" switch under the dashboard that will prevent your car from starting (this can be done by any car alarm company).

  Make your car easier to identify. Place a bright, colorful and unique bumper sticker or applique in a visible location on the back or purchase a personalized license plate from your state Department of Motor Vehicles. If the car disappears you'll want to include this feature when describing the car to authorities.

Elopement "Triggers"

Certain items left around the house can be associated with leaving the house, travel, visiting, taking a walk, etc. By removing them from sight or at the very least not placing them close to the door, you can remove the very reminders that can lead to your loved one leaving the house. Such items may include:

the pet's leash	boots	a lunch box
keys	hats	a brief case
coats or jackets	an umbrella	a suitcase
or even a road map lying on a table		

There are other items that hold important qualities of personal attachment that your loved one would not leave home without. Such items might include her cane, purse, wallet, keys, shoes, glasses, etc. One gentleman we heard about would not leave home without his blanket.

By storing these items in a secure location and out of sight, you may also be creating a passive means of preventing your loved one from leaving home.

"My mom had a purple cape. I don't know whether seeing the cape was the trigger, or if she simply felt "dressed" for a journey when she had it, but when mom had that cape on, she was going!"

K. Deveau, Caregiver

Home Modifications

There are many steps that you can take to protect your loved one and create a safer environment for someone with Alzheimer's disease. There are so many that I have written an entire book on the topic. So rather than add to the length of this book, please let me refer you to *The Complete Guide to Alzheimer's-Proofing Your Home* (Purdue University Press).

This book describes strategies and products to prevent wandering and alert the caregiver of attempts to elope. It can be purchased at The Alzheimer's Store (www.alzstore.com) or by calling (800) 752-3238.

Home modification suggestions include:

- Limit the distance that your loved one can travel:

  install gates and fences;

  use diversions.

- At night, hide or camouflage doorways (use mirrors, curtains, etc.).

- Use devices to alert the caregiver of attempts to elope.

- Secure the home at night to prevent attempts by your loved one to leave while others are asleep. Use locks on doors and door alarms. Locate these locks either up high or down low, outside of the normal field of vision.

Be aware that in the event of a fire or other emergency, locks can hinder safe escape. Never use locks that require keys to unlock them (keys tend to disappear).

NOTES

_____

_____

_____

_____

_____

_____

_____

_____

_____

_____

_____

Wander-Alerting Devices

There are several types of products that will help you discover and prevent a loved one from eloping. Some may even help you find her, if she does manage to get out of the door.

Categories include:

Door alarms and motion detectors

Perimeter and distance monitors

Automatic dialers

Selective alarms and door locking devices

Trackable wander-alert systems

GPS wander alerting devices

**Don't overlook the value of alarms that detect
and notify the caregiver of attempts to elope—**
before your loved one gets out the door.

Door Alarms and Motion Detectors

For those who are in the earliest stages of the disease, the best strategy is to prepare for the future and put in place devices that can notify the in-house caregiver (a spouse, significant other or family member living with the person) of any attempt to approach or open an exit door, especially at night (while others are asleep).

These include door alarms that attach to the door and screech loudly if the door is opened. Though inexpensive, their primary weakness is that they are very loud and startling, and they sound only at the site of violation (the door).

Next are motion detectors that sound an alert when they detect movement approaching or en route to the door (perhaps located in a hallway or foyer). They too sound at the site of violation, but many have options that allow them to sound a melody versus a blood-curdling alarm. However, for those who sleep soundly, there remains no assurance that they will hear or recognize the melodious alert that your loved one is headed for the door.

A step up are door alarms or motion detectors which transmit a signal to a remote receiver (alarm) located elsewhere in the home—perhaps in the caregiver's room. Remember, it is not the person walking out the door that needs to know about it—it is the caregiver (who is likely somewhere else in the home). These alarms can be relatively effective, especially when combined with door locks or other obstacles to leaving the home.

Perimeter and Distance Monitors

There are also more sophisticated devices that require the patient to wear a special bracelet or watch-like transmitter which continuously communicates with a base unit (the receiver). If the transmitter exceeds a pre-programmed distance from the base unit, for example 50 feet, or they violate a defined perimeter (the home or yard) an alarm sounds.

Automatic Phone Dialers

Some of these perimeter and distance monitors can also activate an automatic dialer that will call multiple numbers and provide a pre-recorded emergency message that "Mom has left her building (home, yard, etc.)." For those who live close by, this can provide some peace of mind. But remember, even a person with Alzheimer's can disappear in a matter of seconds—and it often takes much more than that for a distant caregiver to get in the car and drive several blocks (or miles).

Selective Alarms and Door-Locking Devices

Many nursing homes and assisted living facilities employ alarms or automatic door locks that react to approaching bracelets (transmitters) worn by at-risk residents. Though relatively effective, these devices can still be outsmarted (for example, by a gentleman holding the door open for a lady, unaware that she is an Alzheimer's resident); and most are relatively expensive.

Trackable Wander-Alert Systems

Next on the hierarchy are trackable wander-alerting devices. These are perimeter or distance monitoring devices that use a directional radio signal to "point" in the direction of the eloping person (who is wearing the transmitter bracelet). They are limited to a range of about one mile on the ground (less in dense urban settings) and up to five miles when the receiver is used from a helicopter.

GPS Wander Alerting Devices

Finally come the GPS (Global Positioning Satellite) systems that advertise that they can find wanderers and provide their precise location to within a few feet.

GPS tracking systems use a combination of the U.S. Defense Department's satellite system and cellular communication technologies to calculate and transmit a person's (ground) location. The system is based on a network of 24 solar-powered satellites that orbit about 12,000 miles overhead, each constantly broadcasting a radio signal to the Earth below.

Typically, the person at risk wears a receiver which has both GPS and cellular telephone components. It can be worn as a watch-like device; on the belt; sewn into her clothing; or carried in a fanny-pack, backpack, or purse.

When "asked" for its location (by phone), the receiver seeks tracking signals from at least three of the orbiting satellites, then interpolates the data to determine the receiver's latitude and longitude.

Unfortunately, in my opinion, they do not work well enough to be relied upon to save a person's life. Among the problems yet to be resolved are:

> reasonable battery life,
>
> acceptable battery size and weight,
>
> consistent U.S. area coverage,
>
> penetration of signals through buildings,
>
> performance in dense urban settings, and
>
> possible shutdown by the government (to prevent terrorists from using the GPS navigational technology).

On the bright side, however, there are several companies working very hard to resolve these issues and come up with a reliable, acceptable GPS trackable system for Alzheimer's patients.

For the names of companies that offer wander-alerting devices and products, refer to the list of resources in the back of this workbook.

Redundant Strategies

Given the fact that elopement is a life-threatening event, one strategy to prevent its occurrence may not be enough. So rather than simply installing a single alarm, perhaps also installing a chain lock on the door (exceptionally high or low, out of the immediate field of vision) would be twice as good. And then placing a sheet over the door at night would be even better. (For more ideas refer to *The Complete Guide to Alzheimer's-Proofing Your Home,* available at The Alzheimer's Store (www.alzstore.com or call (800) 752-3238).)

The concept of using redundant strategies serves two purposes:

1. to prevent your loved one from eloping; and
2. to alert the caregiver or other member of the household of attempts to elope.

Redundant strategies might include:

- Door alarms and motion detectors (see page 101);
- A black floor mat in front of the door (possibly perceived as a hole by your loved one);
- A STOP sign posted on the door (or a sign that reads "DO NOT ENTER" or "USE OTHER DOOR")
- Door murals to camouflage the door, making it appear to be a set of pantry or bookshelves;
- Multiple locks on exit doors, each requiring different skills to unlock;
- A washcloth taped over the door lock to hide it;
- Sleigh bells attached to the door that will jingle if it is opened;
- Child-proof doorknob covers;
- A fenced yard with a locked gate beyond the door;
- Outdoor furniture removed or secured so that it cannot be used to climb over fences;
- Multiple latching devices on outside gates (that must be operated simultaneously);
- Neighborhood alerts to notify you in the event that your loved one is seen walking outside by himself;
- Walkways and paths that do not lead directly to gates; and
- Diversions to redirect the person heading for the door:

One family whose father had a habit of getting up at night and heading for the garage to drive away in their car placed their beloved cat's bed by the door leading to the garage. When Dad approached the door he'd see Puffy sleeping in her bed, stop and pet her; she'd begin purring, he'd pet some more, then he'd get tired and go back to bed!

Vulnerability Assessment

This assessment can help determine the vulnerability risk of your loved one.[2] It can be completed by a family member, caregiver, facility staff, or an assessment team and should be reviewed at least annually. For healthcare professionals or teams, each "Area to Assess" should be discussed and a determination made as to whether they believe the individual is at "High Risk," "Low Risk," or "No Risk."

---

2. Modified from The Vulnerability Assessment Form created by Community Living Services, Inc., 111 North University, Fargo, ND 58102, Jim Berglie, (701) 232-3133.

There are two specific "types" of vulnerability to be considered when completing this assessment:

1. If the person is currently missing;
2. If the person is likely to come in contact with law enforcement for any other reason (e.g., the individual has an eating disorder and may take food without paying for it; individual may disrobe or show other inappropriate behavior; etc.).

If the missing person is likely to come in contact with law enforcement for a specific reason, that information should be identified and shared with the law enforcement agent in charge.

Areas to Assess	Sample Questions
1 Being taken advantage of by others	Financial; sexual; property: Is the individual easy to manipulate? How does he respond to threats? What will he do to get/keep a friend?
2 Communication skills	How does he communicate? Can he be understood by the general public (verbal or sign, etc.)? How would you describe his comprehension skills?
3 Concept of time, person, place, distance, money	Does he understand these concepts? What does each one of the concepts mean to him?
4 Safety skills	Can he safely cross a street without assistance? How does he respond to emergencies (first aid, fire, etc.)?
5 Identification card	Does he carry his ID card? Does he often lose his card? Does he use the card for cashing checks?
6 Relays personal information (name, address, tel. no.)	Can he provide accurate and current information? Can he be understood by others?
7 Relays provider name	Can he provide a staff person's name? Can he provide that person's telephone number? Can he provide that person's address?
8 Amount of time individual can be on his own	(Assess at his home and in the community.) How long can he be alone/gone before you would get worried?
9 Risk-taking behavior that is consensual	Does he drink alcoholic beverages? Is he sexually active? Does he date?

Areas to Assess	Sample Questions
10 Risk-taking behavior that is non-consensual	Does he understand the rights of others? Does he understand personal boundaries? Has there been any sexual/physical aggression? Does he respect others and their property?
11 Aggression towards others or their property	Is there a behavior plan in place? What are antecedents?
12 Self-abuse	What are typical reactions when afraid, scared, threatened? What is the degree of self-abuse? Does it require/warrant medical intervention?
13 Emergency medical care/drug intervention	What conditions, e.g., epilepsy, diabetes, heart, pica, etc. might require assistance? What might others see (symptoms)? What are symptoms or side effects of medications he may use? What interactions may occur with medications taken and alcohol?
14 Community mobility	What is loved one's preferred mode of transportation? What other possibilities does he have? Does he independently "choose bus" (or other)? Does he know the correct bus to take to get to desired locations?
15 Prior involvement with law enforcement	Look at instances when loved one was identified as a victim. Look at instances when loved one was identified as a potential perpetrator. What was his disposition?

16 Prior missing episodes	What were the circumstances?
	What was loved one's objective?
	  Why did he leave?
	  What did he want?
	  Where did he go
	What was the outcome of the event?

17 Look at any areas unique to the individual, his family, the provider, recent changes.	
18	
19	
20	

Name _____ Date _____

	Areas to Assess	High Risk	Low Risk	No Risk	Comments
1	Being taken advantage of by others				
2	Communication skills				
3	Concept of time, person, place, distance, money				
4	Safety skills				
5	Identification card				
6	Relays personal information (name, address, tel. no.)				
7	Relays provider name				
8	Amount of time individual can be on his own				
9	Risk-taking behavior that is consensual				
10	Risk-taking behavior that is non-consensual				

	Areas to Assess	High Risk	Low Risk	No Risk	Comments
11	Aggression towards others or their property				
12	Self-abuse				
13	Emergency medical care/drug intervention				
14	Community mobility				
15	Prior involvement with law enforcement				
16	Prior missing episodes				
17	Look at any areas unique to the individual, his family, the provider, and recent changes.				
18					
19					
20					

NOTES

Letters, Forms, and Templates

Letters, Forms, and Templates

If and when it becomes necessary to initiate a search, there are a number of tools that can be very helpful, including a missing person profile, flyers and medical release information forms.

Here are some examples and tools to create your own customized forms, letters, and flyers.

Missing Person Profile

Much different from either the initial information that you give to the 911 operator or the data compiled in this workbook, a missing person's profile is a customized, succinct description of your loved one used by law enforcement personnel. It is usually a single sheet of paper (possibly two-sided) which searchers post in their vehicles or carry with them. These profiles provide the details and unique characteristics that distinguish your loved one from other people on the street or who may be found.

Here is an example of a missing person's profile and a blank form to help you create your own.

> ## Note
>
> Take advantage of the questions asked in this workbook.
>
> Highlight information that might be helpful in identifying and finding your loved one.
>
> Include key items in your missing persons profile.
>
> Share the information with law enforcement personnel.

MISSING PERSON PROFILE[1]
(SAMPLE)

Name: Stella Mallory Dickerman

Physical Description:

- 83 years old (appears to most people to be in her 70's or even 60's)
- Height: 5'-3"–5'-5"
- Noticeably rounded shoulders from osteoporosis
- Gray hair (received a permanent on Aug. 28)
- Brown/green eyes (hazel)
- Right-handed
- Excellent teeth, small chip off front tooth
- Black mole in middle of back
- Round black scar—middle of left lower leg
- Recent cut—middle of right lower leg

---

1. *Gone . . . Without a Trace,* Marianne Dickerman Caldwell, Elder Books, Forest Knolls, CA, 1995, pp. 72–74.

- Mild rheumatoid arthritis affecting her back, hands, and right wrist
- Wearing navy blue skirt, white blouse, white sweater, powder blue wind-breaker jacket, tan shoes with laces
- Was carrying a distinctive walking stick (cane) with Alpine decorations (metal markings)

Behavior and Mannerisms:
- Suffers from Alzheimer's disease
- Gentle, trusting, friendly. Readily asks for help. Appreciative of help
- Likes to talk, but confuses words. Forgets what she is saying. Disjointed conversations. Constantly changes topics. Might not be able to give full name or address. Significantly confused about time
- Easily becomes lost
- Packs and repacks suitcases or anything else. Frequently changes clothes
- Likes to walk and can walk long distances

Conversation Topics:
- Her family (son, William; daughter, Marianne; son, Bob or Robert)
- Her parents (her father, who died suddenly of the flu; her mother who operated a college dormitory called "The Vatican" in Oberlin, Ohio, or Oberlin College)
- Country school
- Water-color painting (she was an artist)
- Battle Creek, Michigan or Chatauqua Lake, New York

Please notify Police or Sheriff's Department (name)

_____

Tel. no. (_____) _____

List the names of two family members and their telephone numbers:

_____ (_____) _____

_____ (_____) _____

NOTES

_____

_____

_____

_____

_____

_____

Missing Person Profile *(continued)*

MISSING PERSON PROFILE

Last Updated: _____

Name		Nickname:
Age:	Height:	Weight:
Hair color:	Sex:	Date missing:
Race:	Language spoken:	

Description (general appearance, eye color, hair description, unique physical features)

_____

_____

_____

_____

_____

Clothing Last Seen Wearing

_____

_____

_____

Point Last Seen and Conditions of Disappearance

_____

_____

_____

_____

_____

Behavior & Mannerisms

_____

_____

_____

_____

❏ Suffers from Alzheimer's disease

General disposition:

_____

_____

_____

_____

Subject may be looking for:

_____

_____

_____

_____

Subject may be attracted to:

_____

_____

_____

_____

Favorite Topics of Conversation

_____

_____

_____

_____

Items That May Be in Person's Possession

_____

_____

Missing Person Profile *(continued)*

Medical Conditions

_____

_____

_____

_____

Please notify Police or Sheriff's Department (name) _____

Tel. no. (_____) _____

Family Member	Tel. No.	Cell Phone No.

Status: <u>MISSING AT RISK, MEDICALLY ENDANGERED ELDER</u>

What other features, mannerisms or behaviors would distinguish your loved one from other people on the street?

_____

_____

_____

_____

_____

What additional information would you like to include in your missing person's profile?

_____

_____

_____

Missing Person's Flyer

Among the steps you will also want to take if your loved one is not found within a reasonable time is to enroll the eyes and ears of the community. Among the best ways to do this are to engage the media (radio, TV, and newspapers) and to put up and hand out flyers. Teenagers volunteering to help can be a valuable means of distributing these flyers.

Here's a sample of a missing person's flyer.[2]

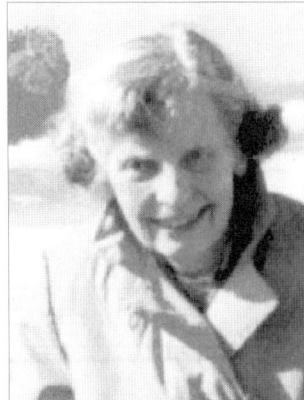

MISSING
Since September 13,1991

STELLA MALLORY DICKERMAN is an 83-year-old woman with Alzheimer's disease, 5'-4," 112 lbs, gray hair, hazel eyes.

If you find any of the following items, or have any information, please contact:

Rindge Police Department :
Tel. (000) 000-0000

- Wooden walking cane with metal Australian shields & "OZT" engraved on top
- Woman's light "sky blue" windbreaker jacket
- Tan shoes & navy blue skirt
- White sweater & white blouse
- Noticeably rounded shoulders from osteoporosis

Stella was last seen at a children's softball game at a boarding school outside of Rindge, New Hampshire. There is a possibility that she accepted a ride out of the area.

2. This is a sample missing person's flyer used by the family of Stella Mallory Dickerman. Source: *Gone . . . Without a Trace,* Marianne Dickerman Caldwell, Elder Books, Forest Knolls, CA, 1995. Reprinted with permission.

NCIC Missing Person Report Form
(National Crime Information Center—Refer also to information on page 136)

The FBI National Crime Information Center (NCIC) is the nation's primary database for information on missing persons. The following document is the standard form used by the NCIC to describe people who have been reported missing and are the subjects of ongoing searches. The format is often used as the basis for law enforcement forms, missing person profiles, and reports. Use it to help you create and compile information about your loved one that will help authorities identify or distinguish her from other people walking around in public.

NOTES

_____

_____

_____

_____

_____

_____

_____

_____

_____

_____

_____

_____

_____

_____

_____

_____

_____

_____

_____

_____

_____

_____

_____

_____

MISSING PERSON REPORT FOR NCIC RECORD ENTRY

Message Key (MKE)	Reporting Agency (ORI)	Name of Missing Person (NAM)
☐ Disability (EMD) ☐ Juvenile(EMJ) ☐ Endangered (EME) ☐ Victim (EMV) ☐ Involuntary (EMI) ☐ Caution		

Sex (SEX)	Race (RAC)	Place of Birth (POB)	Date of Birth (DOB)	Date of Emancipation (DOE)
☐ Male (M) ☐ Female (F)	Race ☐ Asian or Pacific Islander (A) ☐ Unknown (U) ☐ Black ☐ White ☐ American Indian. Alaskan Native (I)			

Height (HGT)	Weight (WGT)	Eye Color (EYE)	Hair Color (HAI)	FBI Number (FBI)
		☐ Black (BLK) ☐ Hazel (HAZ) ☐ Blue (BLU) ☐ Maroon (MAR) ☐ Brown (BRO) ☐ Multicolored (MUL) ☐ Gray (GRY) ☐ Pink (PNK) ☐ Green (GRN) ☐ Unknown (XXX)	Hair Color ☐ Black (BLK) ☐ Brown (BRO) ☐ Blonde/Strawberry (BLN) ☐ Gray/Partially Gray (GRY) ☐ Red/Auburn (RED) ☐ White (WHI) ☐ Sandy (SDY) ☐ Unknown (XXX)	

Skin Tone (SKN)	Scars, marks, tattoos, and other characteristics (SMT)	Fingerprint Classification (FPC)
☐ Albino ☐ Olive (OLV) ☐ Black (BLK) ☐ Ruddy (RDY) ☐ Dark (DRK) ☐ Sallow (SAL) ☐ Dk Brown (DBR) ☐ Yellow (YEL) ☐ Fair (FAR) ☐ Light (LGT) ☐ Lt. Brown (LBR) ☐ Medium (MED) ☐ Med. Brown (MBR)		

Other Identifying Numbers (MNP)	Social Security Number (SOC)	Operator's License Number (OLN)	Operator's License State (OLB)	Operator's License Year of Expiration (OLY)

Missing Person (MNP)	Date of Last Contact (DLC)	Originating Agency Case Number (OCA)	Miscellaneous (MIS)
☐ Missing Person (MP) ☐ Catastrophe Victim (DV)			Include build, handedness, any illness or diseases, clothing description, hair description, etc.

Miscellaneous Information

MISSING PERSON REPORT FOR NCIC RECORD ENTRY *(continued)*

Below is a list of clothing and personal effects. Please indicate those items the missing person was last seen wearing. Include style, type, color, labels or laundry markings. (MIS)

Item	Style/Type	Size	Color	Markings	Item	Style/Type	Size	Color	Markings
Head Gear					Shoes/Boots/Sneakers				
Scarf/Tie/Gloves					Underwear				
Coat/Jacket/Vest					Bra/Girdle/Slip				
Sweater					Stockings/Pantyhose				
Shirt/Blouse					Wallet/Purse				
Pants/Skirt					Money				
Belts/Suspenders					Glasses				
Socks					Other				

LICENSE PLATE AND VEHICLE INFORMATION

License Plate Number (LIC)   State (LIS)   Year Expires (LIY)   License Plate Type (LIT)

Vehicle Identification Number (VIN)   Year (VYR)   Make (VMA)   Model (VMO)   Style (VST)   Color (VCO)

Does the missing person have corrected vision? (SMT) ☐ Yes Where? ____ Has missing person ever donated blood? ☐ No ☐ Yes Where?   Has the missing person ever been fingerprinted? ☐ No ☐ Yes If so, by whom?

Blood Type
☐ A Positive (APOS)   ☐ B Positive (BPOS)
☐ A Negative (ANEG)   ☐ B Negative (BNEG)
☐ A Unknown (AUNK)   ☐ B Unknown (BUNK)
☐ O Positive (OPOS)   ☐ AB Positive (ABPOS)
☐ O Negative (ONEG)   ☐ AB Negative (ABNEG)
☐ O Unknown (OUNK)   ☐ AB Unknown (ABUNK)   (BLT)

Circumcision (CRC)
☐ Was (C)   Unknown (U)
☐ Was Not (N)

Footprints available (FPA)
☐ Yes (Y)
☐ No (N)

Body X-Rays (BXR)
☐ Full (F)   ☐ None (N)
☐ Partial

Corrective Vision Prescription   Jewelry Type (VRX)   Jewelry Description (JWT)   (JWL)

Aliases   Reporting Agency Telephone Number   Reporting Officer

Complainant's Name   Complainant's Address   Complainant's Telephone Number

Relationship of Complainant to Missing Person   Missing Person's Address   Missing Person's Occupation (MIS)

NCIC Number (NIC)   Places missing person frequented

Close friends/relatives   Possible destination

Investigating Officer and Telephone Number (MIS)   Complainant's signature

Medical Information Release Form

In order for your dentist or physician to release confidential medical information to officials involved in the search for your loved one, a medical information release form (next page) will need to be signed by your loved one or her legal guardian.

Have this form ready and available in the event that information contained in her medical records is needed to help find your loved one or to make a positive identification.

It would be wise to fill out copies of this form and give them to your dentist and physician to keep in your loved one's file, just in case it might one day be needed. If you are the legal guardian for your loved one, include copies of the documentation.

This can save a lot of time and trouble in the event that law enforcement needs a copy of your loved one's medical information.

NOTES

_____

_____

_____

_____

_____

_____

_____

_____

_____

_____

_____

_____

_____

_____

_____

_____

_____

_____

_____

_____

AUTHORIZATION TO RELEASE PATIENT INFORMATION

Patient Name _____ Date of Birth _____

Patient Soc. Sec. # _____

I hereby authorize and request:

Physician/Medical Office _____

    Address _____

    City _____ State _____ Zip _____

Telephone Number (_____) _____

to disclose All Patient Information and Medical Records to the following individual or organization:

Police/Sheriff's Dept. _____

    Address _____

    City _____ State _____ Zip _____

Telephone Number (_____) _____

I understand that the information in my health record may include information relating to communicable disease, Acquired Immunodeficiency Syndrome ("AIDS"), or Human Immunodeficiency Virus ("HIV"), behavioral or mental health, alcohol/drug(substance) abuse or any such related information.

Description of the purpose of the use and/or disclosure:

____ Continuing Care   ____ Second Opinion   ____ Social Security/Disability

____ Consultation   ____ Insurance   ____ Legal purposes

____ Personal Use   ✓ Other: Patient Identification or other use by law enforcement personnel.

____ I understand that this authorization is voluntary and I may refuse to sign this authorization.

____ I understand I may inspect or copy the information to be used or disclosed.

____ I understand I may revoke this authorization at any time by notifying the doctor listed above in writing.

____ I understand that information used or disclosed pursuant to the authorization may be subject to redisclosure by the recipient and may no longer be protected by federal and state privacy regulations.

This authorization will be in effect until _____ (date).

_____   _____
  Signature of Patient or Patient's Representative   Date

_____
Printed name of Patient or Patient's Representative

_____ or _____
     Relationship to Patient   Legal Authority *(attach supporting documentation)*

Letter to the Medical Examiner or Coroner

Certainly, we hope this workbook is never needed, but if and when, despite everyone's best efforts, your loved one is not found within 48 hours, it may become prudent to check with local medical examiners and coroner offices. Call them for their address or fax number. You can find their telephone number under the county listings in your telephone book or by calling "Information" (411).

A letter such as this, sent to your county medical examiner or coroner (and those in surrounding counties), allows them to notify law enforcement officials and inform you in the event that the descriptions of your loved one do or do not match any of their unidentified deceased victims.

Here is an example of the type of letter you should send:[1]

It is also a good idea to include a self-addressed, stamped postcard and a photo of your loved one.

```
To:    Office of County Medical Examiner
       (Address)

From:  (Name )
       (Address)
       (City, State, Zip Code)
       (Phone)

Re:    Unidentified Body

I am writing with regard to my mother, Stella Mallory Dickerman,
an eighty-three year old Alzheimer's disease victim who vanished
on September 13, 1991.
    She walked away from a children's softball game at a school lo-
cated outside of Rindge, New Hampshire. The school is situated ap-
proximately one mile from the New Hampshire-Massachusetts border.
    Despite an extensive search, immediately launched, of the area
surrounding the school, no clues have surfaced and she remains un-
found. There is a possibility that she may have been given a
ride and dropped off outside of the area, met with foul play or
died from exposure.
    I have enclosed a self-addressed postcard for you to note your
findings. I can be reached at the phone number listed above for ad-
ditional information.
    Thank you very much for your help in this matter.

Sincerely,

Marianne Dickerman Caldwell
```

1. *Gone . . . Without a Trace,* Marianne Dickerman Caldwell, Elder Books, Forest Knolls, CA, 1995, pp. 76–77.

Identification Cards

Fill out these ID Cards. Cut them out and place one in your loved one's wallet/purse and in other locations where she might be discovered if she were found wandering by herself.

I.D. CARD

Name _____

Address _____

City, State, Zip: _____

In case of emergency, please notify:

Name _____

Tel. No. (_____) _____

Cell Ph. No. (_____) _____

I.D. CARD

Name _____

Address _____

City, State, Zip: _____

In case of emergency, please notify:

Name _____

Tel. No. (_____) _____

Cell Ph. No. (_____) _____

I.D. CARD

Name _____

Address _____

City, State, Zip: _____

In case of emergency, please notify:

Name _____

Tel. No. (_____) _____

Cell Ph. No. (_____) _____

I.D. CARD

Name _____

Address _____

City, State, Zip: _____

In case of emergency, please notify:

Name _____

Tel. No. (_____) _____

Cell Ph. No. (_____) _____

I.D. CARD

Name _____

Address _____

City, State, Zip: _____

In case of emergency, please notify:

Name _____

Tel. No. (_____) _____

Cell Ph. No. (_____) _____

I.D. CARD

Name _____

Address _____

City, State, Zip: _____

In case of emergency, please notify:

Name _____

Tel. No. (_____) _____

Cell Ph. No. (_____) _____

I.D. CARD

Name _____

Address _____

City, State, Zip: _____

In case of emergency, please notify:

Name _____

Tel. No. (_____) _____

Cell Ph. No. (_____) _____

I.D. CARD

Name _____

Address _____

City, State, Zip: _____

In case of emergency, please notify:

Name _____

Tel. No. (_____) _____

Cell Ph. No. (_____) _____

Part 10

Programs

Programs

In the field of Alzheimer's and finding people with the disease who might be lost, there are important programs that you should know about. Some train the first responders about Alzheimer's disease, while others provide valuable information that can contribute to your loved one's safe return in the event she is discovered missing.

The Safe Return Program

For anyone prone to wandering, we highly recommend the Alzheimer's Association's Safe Return Program. Safe Return has facilitated the recovery of more than 10,000 people with Alzheimer's disease to their families and caregivers with over a 99 percent rate of success.

The Alzheimer's Association Safe Return Program is a national, government-funded program that assists in the identification and safe, timely return of individuals with Alzheimer's disease and related dementias who wander off and become lost.

The program includes:

- Identification wallet cards, jewelry, clothing labels, lapel pin, and bag tags;
- A national photo/information database;
- A 24-hour toll-free emergency crisis line;
- Alzheimer's Association local chapter support; and
- Wandering behavior education and training for caregivers and families.

If the registrant wanders and is found, the person who finds him can call the Safe Return toll-free number located on the wanderer's identification wallet card, bracelet, or clothing labels. The Safe Return telephone operator will then immediately alert the family members or caregiver listed in the database, so they can be reunited with their loved one.

When registering online or by phone, you will be asked to provide the following information:

- Registrant's name and contact information;
- Registrant's identifying characteristics (Social Security number, height, weight, eye color, distinguishing marks and characteristics, etc.);
- Registrant's exact wrist measurement in inches (required when ordering a bracelet);
- Up to three contact names, addresses, and phone numbers;
- Local law enforcement information (address, phone, and fax numbers); and
- Credit card number and expiration date

On the front of the bracelet it simply says:

Safe Return

On the back of the bracelet it says:

MEMORY IMPAIRED

To help _____ (First Name)

Call 1-800-572-1122

I.D. # _____

(Safe Return bracelets are also available for the caregiver that say, "I am a caregiver for _____.")

The cost of enrollment in the Safe Return Program is a one-time fee of $40.00. The jewelry costs an additional $5.00. Check with your local Alzheimer's Association chapter to find out if grants are available in your area to cover the cost of enrollment.

For more information or to register in the Safe Return Program go to http://www.alz.org/Services/SafeReturn.asp or call (888) 572-8566.

> Note also that many local Alzheimer's organizations have ID bracelet programs which are coordinated with local Police or Sheriff's Departments. It would be worthwhile to call your local Alzheimer's organization to inquire.

The Safely Home Program (Canada)

In Canada you can register your loved one with the Safely Home™ Alzheimer Wandering Registry, a nationwide program designed to help find persons with Alzheimer's who are lost and assist in their safe return home. Developed by the Alzheimer Society of Canada in partnership with the Royal Canadian Mounted Police, the registry stores vital information confidentially on a law enforcement database. The information can be accessed by law enforcement anywhere in Canada and the United States.

For a one-time registration fee of $25, the Safely Home Program provides you with an identification bracelet, a caregiver handbook, and ID cards. Having your loved one wear the bracelet and keeping the cards in your loved one's wallet, purse, and coat pocket can aid in quickly identifying him should he become lost.

For more information contact your local Alzheimer's Society chapter office, call (800) 616-8816 or go to http://www.alzheimer.ca/english/safelyhome/intro.htm.

Local Alzheimer's Organization Wanderer ID Programs

Though the Alzheimer's Association's Safe Return Program is an excellent program with a proven record of success, you should not overlook local Alzheimer's organizations which may also have wanderer ID programs. Call your local Alzheimer's organization or resource center to inquire if they have a wanderer ID bracelet program and ask about other services they offer.

Community Alzheimer's Alert Programs

A small number of law enforcement departments around the country have their own Alzheimer's Alert Program whereby families living in the community who care for a loved one with Alzheimer's disease can register their loved one.

With these programs, in the event that this person becomes missing the local police or sheriff's department already has her picture and information on file and the search can begin immediately. Or if the individual is found and unable to tell them where she lives (even with no missing person's report filed), they can identify her through an on-file photograph.

Here are some examples of such programs. Please feel free to contact these pioneers, inquire about their programs, and work with them and your local law enforcement organization to create an Alzheimer's Alert Program for your community.

Title	Jurisdiction	Contact Information
Alzheimer's Alert Program	Cumberland, RI	Sgt. Michael L. Kinch (401) 333-2500
Alzheimer's Alert Program	Marshfield, MA	Sgt. Paul Taber (781) 834-6655 (ext. 230)
Alzheimer's Alert Program	Norwood, MA	Lt. Brian P. Murphy (781) 762-1212 bmurphy@ci.norwood.ma.us
Wanderer Assist Program	Lynn Haven, FL	Capt. Matt Riemer (850) 265-4111 policedept@cityoflynnhaven.com
Wanderer's Identification Program	Collier County, FL	Maggie Straub (239) 262-8388
W.A.S.P. (Wandering Adult Service and Protection)	Versailles, KY	Chief Allen Love (859) 873-3126 info@versaillesky.com

This is surely not a complete list of all local Alzheimer's Alert Programs. We apologize if we have failed to include your community's program. Please contact us at AgelessD@aol.com to be included in future editions of *In Search of the Alzheimer's Wanderer.*

The Atlanta "Mattie's Call" Alert System
On April 21, 2004, Mattie Moore, a 68 year-old Alzheimer's patient, wandered away from her home in Atlanta, GA. Her body was not found until December 25, 2004.

As a result, in June 2004, the Atlanta City Council formally adopted an emergency alert system named "Mattie's Call" to help find missing Alzheimer's patients.

With the "Mattie's Call" Alert System, if a person with Alzheimer's is missing, the family can call the Atlanta Police. Information on the missing person will then be announced on the radio, TV, on freeway signs, and other systems, similar to an Amber Alert for children. Their hope is to expand this system to all of Georgia and then to the nation.

For more information on the Mattie's Call Alert System call Alice Hoffmann at the Atlanta Alzheimer's Association office at (404) 728-1181.

Project Lifesaver
Project Lifesaver is a national program that provides trackable bracelets to families and communities. Units can be sold to individuals caring for a loved one with Alzheimer's disease or furnished to communities through sponsored donations. Sensitive tracking receivers are provided to member law enforcement jurisdictions.

Each bracelet has its own frequency and emits a signal which can be located by a receiver (mounted in a police vehicle or helicopter). Project Lifesaver also works with local law enforcement to help find lost wanderers and trains police personnel to use the equipment and conduct the program.

In addition, families can purchase compatible distance monitoring alarms that will alert caregivers when their loved one, wearing the bracelet, wanders beyond a pre-programmed distance from a base unit located within the home. Portable, hand-held tracking receivers are also available that will "point" in the direction of the missing person up to a mile away.

Project Lifesaver has completed over 1,200 successful search and rescue missions for wandering victims of Alzheimer's disease, autism, Down's syndrome and dementia-related disorders. All persons were found alive and returned home—most within a half hour.

Contact your local police or sheriff's department to see if they participate in the Project Lifesaver Program or contact Project Lifesaver at (757) 546-5502.

NOTES

NOTES

Part 11

Tools for Law Enforcement

Tools for Law Enforcement

The goal of any search is to find the missing person quickly and to return him home to his family and loved ones healthy.

The following information is designed for law enforcement personnel by experts in the field of law enforcement and Alzheimer's. It offers:

- strategical fine tuning to assess the urgency of the search,
- guidelines based on the amount of time elapsed since the person was discovered missing,
- steps and recommended resources, and
- additional information for comprehensive searches suited to the unique demands imposed by Alzheimer's disease.

Alzheimer's and Related Disorders Missing Person Checklist[1]

This is a general checklist for law enforcement agencies when responding to a missing person report involving a subject with Alzheimer's or a related memory impairment. An aggressive law enforcement response is required to protect life due to the high urgency of searches for people with Alzheimer's and related disorders. As with any general checklist, some items may not apply, additional steps may be required, and the order may be changed.

Dispatch

- Determine name, address, call-back number, relationship to missing subject.
- Determine age, medical conditions, special disabilities of missing subject.
- Caller's reason for reporting the subject missing.
- Dispatch an officer/deputy.

Initial Report Collection

- Name, nicknames, aliases, age, race, gender of missing subject.
- Whether the person can communicate, knows own name and address, or can speak English.
- Place (address), date, time, circumstances of when subject was last seen.
- Last seen by whom, and how to contact that person.
- Complete physical description, including clothing.
- Whether the person is carrying any ID, money, credit or ATM cards, or other items.
- Whether the missing person is registered with *Safe Return* and wearing any program items (bracelet, necklace, clothing labels, or wallet ID.)
- Summary of physical and mental health, including medications.
- History of subject, past wandering, previous searches, where found.
- Determine whether subject is on foot or using other transportation (public or private).
- Initial actions taken by caller.

Initial Officer/Deputy Actions

- Collect initial report.
- Determine degree of physical search warranted.

---

1. This checklist was produced with the support and collaboration of The Virginia Center of Aging Grant 97-02 to Robert J. Koester, the Virginia Department of Emergency Services, and the Virginia Search and Rescue Council. Version 1.5, March 3, 2001.

If a physical search is warranted:

- Identify and secure the Point Last Seen (PLS) or Last Known Position (LKP) as a crime scene.
- Place barrier tape.
- Secure scent article.
- Secure tracks.
- Remove or stop idling engines.
- Contact shift supervisor and/or SAR coordinator, request additional resources.
- Search residence and grounds if applicable, regardless of previous efforts.
- Patrol immediate area.

Shift Supervisor/SAR Coordinator Actions

- Receive initial report from initial officer/deputy.
- Implement initial command structure.
- Determine urgency of search efforts (see Search Urgency Checklist.)
- Determine initial resource needs.

Suggested Guidelines for Resource Deployment*
(Refer to Search Urgency Evaluation Checklist page 134 to evaluate and determine level of urgency.)

Emergency Search	**High Urgency**	**Moderate Urgency**
Initial Search	*Initial Search*	*Initial Search*
Add'l. law enforcement	Add'l. law enforcement	Add'l. law enforcement
Investigator	Investigator	Investigator
Local tracking dogs	Local tracking dogs	Local tracking dogs
Helicopter (FLIR)	Helicopter (FLIR)	Helicopter (FLIR)
Local SAR resources	Local SAR resources	Local SAR resources
Local Fire/Rescue		
After 0–2 hours*	*After 2–6 hours**	*After 4–12 hours**
Search management	Search management	Search management
(Overhead Team)	(Overhead Team)	(Overhead Team)
Trained field teams	Trained field teams	Trained field teams
Trained team leaders	Trained team leaders	Trained team leaders
Tracking dogs	Tracking dogs	Tracking dogs
Air-scent dogs	Air-scent dogs	Air-scent dogs
Mantrackers	Mantrackers	Mantrackers
Horses, bike	Horses, bike	Horses, bike
Fixed wings	Fixed wings	Fixed wings
PIO	Local Fire/Rescue	Local Fire/Rescue
Logistical support	Logistical support	Logistical support

*These are only suggested guidelines for resource deployment. Localities may choose a more aggressive response or limit resource requests based upon each unique search.

Further actions include:

- Establish location of search base or staging area for incoming resources.
- Notify Department of Emergency Management.
- Request or alert specialized resources.
- Contact the Alzheimer's Association Safe Return Program (800) 572-1122 and your local Wanderer's ID program (if applicable).
- Obtain photograph of subject and prepare information flyer.
- Issue radio report to surrounding jurisdictions.
- Enter subject into NCIC Network.
- Contact local hospitals (Emergency Room and Psychiatric Ward).
- Contact local transportation hubs.
- Contact emergency services agencies.
- Contact local shelters.
- Contact morgues and medical examiners' office.
- Determine search area (theoretical, statistical, subjective, deductive).
- Deploy initial reflex tasks:

    — Highly systematic search of residence/nursing home and grounds by law enforcement.
    — Send patrols to areas the subject has been previously located.
    — Investigative task of canvassing neighborhood.
    — Patrols along roads.
    — Establish containment points.
    — Tracking dogs from PLS and along roadways.
    — Mantrackers from PLS.
    — Deploy air-scent dog teams into drainages and streams, starting nearest PLS.
    — Early deployment of hasty ground teams into drainages and streams nearest the PLS.
    — Cut for sign along roadways.
    — Dog teams and ground sweep teams (in separate sectors) expanding from PLS. Ensure teams search heavy briars/bushes.
    — Air-scent dog teams and ground sweep teams tasked 100 yards (initially) parallel to roadways.
    — Search nearby previous home sites and the region between home sites and PLS.
    — Repeat search of residence/nursing home grounds at least twice a day.
    — Post flyers in appropriate locations.

- Notify change of shifts within own department/office.
- Ask neighboring law enforcement agencies to include a report in all shift briefings.
- Notify local postal officials.
- Inform media if:

    — Missing person has a life-threatening health problem, such as insulin-dependent diabetes.
    — Weather is extreme.
    — It is dark out, the person has been missing for more than two hours, and an active search effort is ongoing.

SAR Incident Commander Actions

The precise order of tasks upon arrival will change depending upon the unique circumstances of the search. The IC must be highly flexible during the first hours of an incident. The following list serves as a suggestion for initial tasks. The precise order of these steps will vary from incident to incident. This list should not be considered inclusive.

- Appoint investigations and operations chief (OPS) from most qualified individuals present and allow them to begin their jobs. Activate other elements of the Incident Command System (ICS) as needed.

- Delegate sign-in procedure to competent individual.

- Brief command and general staff.

- Consider moving base if minimum base requirements are not met at current location:

  — Electricity, lights (generator may provide).
  — Work area sheltered from weather, media, family.
  — Telephone and copier (if not brought).
  — Radio communications (if not established).
  — Staging area, sanitation, running water, and parking area if large search.

- Determine information needs and inform applicable personnel of needs.

- Develop initial objectives/strategies (develop or delegate tactics).

- Coordinate staff activity, manage incident.

- If appropriate, ensure that operations is developing tasks and dispatching teams within 30 minutes of arrival.

- Determine OPS needs for any resources.

- Approve the use of different training levels on the incident.

- Ensure efficient flow of personnel from staging area to field.

- Identify and meet with liaisons/agency representatives to keep informed and determine their special capabilities and requirements.

- Work to create an environment for staff to work in, i.e., get things done. Shield staff from family, media, and political pressures.

- Verify that everyone on general staff is being kept up-to-date.

- Establish parameters for general staff members to increase staffing levels.

- Ensure tentative medical/evacuation plan developed in conjunction with local EMS/Rescue.

- Ensure staff meeting documentation requirements (investigative folder, task completed map, debriefing logs, clue map, clue log, communication log, unit logs).

- Evaluate logistical needs, future needs, and ensure they will be met.

Search Urgency Evaluation

Weather Profile	Values
Recent past and/or short term forecast for severe weather	1
Forecast for severe weather within 8 hours or less	1–2
Forecast for severe weather more than 8 hours away	2
No forecast for severe weather	3
Location Terrain/Hazard Profile	
Known hazards in the area or difficult terrain in suspected area	1
Few or no known hazards in the area	2
Age	
Age greater than 65	1
Age 65 or less	2
Medical Condition	
Known or suspected illness, injury, or memory problems	1
Known or suspected fatality (i.e., drowning, suicide)	3
Number of Subjects in Party	
One person out alone or with another Alzheimer's patient	1
Alzheimer's subject lost with someone of normal cognitive ability	2–3
Subject Preparedness Profile	
Inadequate equipment and clothing for environment and weather	1
Questionable equipment and clothing for environment and weather	2
Subject Experience Profile	
Not experienced outdoors and does not know the area	1
Not experienced, but remembers the area	2
Recalls outdoors experience and does not know the area	3
Recalls outdoors experience, and remembers the area	4

TOTAL *(Add up applicable values in right column)*

Emergency Search = 7–12   **High Urgency = 13–17**   **Moderate Urgency = 18–19**

Any search for an Alzheimer's disease subject in poor weather should be considered an EMERGENCY search. Any search for a known fatality is MODERATE to LOW urgency.

References

Flaherty, G. (1995) *Law Enforcement, Alzheimer's Disease & the Lost Elder.* Cambridge, MA: Alzheimer's Association.

Koester, R. (1996) *Field Operations Guide for Search & Rescue.* Charlottesville, VA: dbS Productions.

Koester, R., and Stooksbury, D. (1992) Lost subject profile of Alzheimer's. *Journal of Search, Rescue, and Emergency Response* 11(4): 20–26.

Search and Rescue Resource Guide. (1996) Virginia Department of Emergency Services. Richmond, VA.

Police, Fire/Rescue, and Search and Rescue Resources and Training[2]

A Child Is Missing (ACIM)   ACIM is a national program that assists law enforcement and families when a child or elderly (often with Alzheimer's) or disabled person is reported missing.

When notified by the police or sheriff's office, ACIM will collect pertinent information, make a recorded message, and create a database of the telephone numbers of all homes and businesses in the area. This message is then sent out via a high-speed dialing system (1,000 calls in 60 seconds).

ACIM continues to work with the searchers until the missing person is found. At that time ACIM will fax a case follow-up to the officer in charge, documenting the conclusion and results of the search. ACIM's services are free to law enforcement.

For more information on A Child Is Missing Program, call 888-875-2246 or go to www.achildismissing.org.

dbS Productions   An informational resource for Law Enforcement, Fire Rescue, and Search & Rescue personnel with a special focus on finding missing Alzheimer's wanderers.

dbS Productions provides classes, publications, and training aids developed to assist law enforcement and search and rescue planners with regard to finding people with Alzheimer's disease.

To contact dbS go to www.dbS-sar.com; call (800) 745-1581; or write to dbS Productions, P.O. Box 1894, Charlottesville, VA 22903.

Local Alzheimer's Assn. Chapters & Alzheimer's Organizations   Many local Alzheimer's Association chapters and Alzheimer's organizations provide Alzheimer's training for law enforcement officers and other emergency personnel. Contact your local Alzheimer's Association chapter, local Alzheimer's organization, or Alzheimer's resource center to inquire what kind of training they offer.

National Council for Certified Dementia Practitioners (NCCPD)   The NCCDP provides Alzheimer's training to law enforcement and emergency first responders. For more information go to http://www.nccdp.org or call (877) 729-5191.

National Institute for Elopement Prevention and Resolution (NIEPR)   The National Institute for Elopement was developed to assist and educate facilities and families caring for those who suffer from illnesses that debilitate and diminish the individual's ability to care for himself, which can lead to elopements.

NIEPR assists and educates those who update the policies and procedures that govern elopement prevention and response plans. The institute provides consulting, speakers, workshops, facility reviews, elopement response plans, staff training, elopement prevention products, and search and rescue assistance. For more information go to www.elopement.org or call (785) 286-0444.

Project Far From Home   Project Far From Home is a national law-enforcement educational program designed to teach law enforcement and search and rescue teams about missing at-risk Alzheimer's and dementia subjects.

The goal of Project Far From Home is to educate law enforcement officers and other public safety personnel in order to further increase the opportunities to find and return missing persons with Alzheimer's or a related dementia to their loved ones.

To contact Project Far From Home go to www.projectfarfromhome.org; call (760) 315-1895; or e-mail at info@projectfarfromhome.org.

---

2. This checklist was produced with the support and collaboration of the Virginia Center of Aging Grant 97-02 to Robert J. Koester, the Virginia Department of Emergency Services, and the Virginia Search and Rescue Council. Version 1.5, March 3, 2001.

Project Lifesaver   An innovative rapid response program aiding victims and families suffering from Alzheimer's disease and related disorders. By forming partnerships with local law enforcement and public safety organizations, Project Lifesaver deploys specially trained teams with technology to locate wandering adults (wearing trackable bracelets—see pages 75 and 113).

Project Lifesaver works with local law enforcement agencies to provide training, tracking devices, and trackable wristbands for people in the community with Alzheimer's disease.

To contact Project Lifesaver call (757) 546-5502, go to www.projectlifesaver.org, or write to Project Lifesaver, 815 Battlefield Blvd S., Chesapeake, VA 23322.

National Crime Information Center (NCIC) 2000   The FBI National Crime Information Center (NCIC) 2000 is a 24/7 nationwide information system dedicated to serving and supporting criminal justice agencies—local, state, and federal—in their mission to uphold the law and protect the public. NCIC 2000 serves criminal justice agencies in all 50 states, the District of Columbia, the Commonwealth of Puerto Rico, the United States Virgin Islands, and Canada, as well as federal agencies with law enforcement missions.

Typically, the FBI does not become involved in a case unless there is evidence of foul play crossing state lines. However, if your loved one is not found after a reasonable amount of time, it might be wise to request that your loved one's doctor and dentist release medical information to the NCIC in order to better disseminate and facilitate information about your loved one.

This may require the family or legal guardian to fill out a medical release form allowing the missing person's doctor to provide this information (see page 120).

You can call the NCIC at (304) 625-3000, fax the form to (304) 625-5393, or send it to:

National Crime Information Center (NCIC)

Criminal Justice Information Services (CJIS) Division

1000 Custer Hollow Road

Clarksburg, West Virginia 26306

For more information go to:

www.fas.org/irp/agency/doj/fbi/is/ncic.htm

http://www.fbi.gov/hq/cjisd/ncic.htm.

Part 12

Definitions and Acronyms

Definitions and Acronyms

Activities of Daily Living (ADLs)—Basic daily tasks, functions and responsibilities required to maintain one's health, sustenance and independence. The primary activities of daily living are toileting, bathing, dressing, eating, ambulation and continence.

Catastrophic Reactions—Extreme emotional responses seemingly disproportionate to their apparent cause.

Delusions—fixed false beliefs.

Dementia—Often misused as a synonym for Alzheimer's disease or memory loss, dementia means chronic confusion severe enough to interfere with daily life or activities of daily living. More of a symptom than a condition, dementia can be caused by any one of a number of different illnesses, injuries or conditions, including a stroke, Parkinson's, HIV, Pick's Disease (Frontal Lobe Dementia), Huntington's Disease, Creutzfeldt-Jacob Disease, Binswanger Disease, Lewy Body Disease, thyroid disorder, vitamin deficiency, severe head trauma, and others. Dementia can affect memory, judgment, thinking, visual-spatial and communicative skills.

Elopement—(1) the most serious form of wandering whereby a person finds himself outside of the home or attempts to leave the safety of his home, caregivers, or family, unable or unwilling to return. It can be intentional or unintentional; (2) when a patient wanders away, walks away, runs away, escapes, or otherwise leaves a care-giving facility or environment unsupervised, unnoticed, and/or prior to his scheduled discharge.[1]

Fiblets—For a person whose intent and mindset is based upon irrational thought, honesty may not be the best policy. For their own safety, white lies or "fiblets" may be the best course of action.

> YOU: *Hi Beth, where are you going?*
> BETH: *I have to go pick up my children from school.*
> YOU: *Oh, Beth, I just spoke to them on the phone. They're at home.*
>   *They wanted me to tell you that everything is just fine.*

First Responder—refers to any law enforcement officer responding to your call for help, including police and sheriff's departments, fire rescue, emergency rescue personnel, search and rescue, etc.

FLIR—Forward Looking Infrared system is a thermal imaging device designed to be aircraft mounted, usually on a helicopter, that can detect heat sources at night. It's useful in locating persons who may be fleeing on foot, hiding in dense foliage, concealed in vehicles, or huddled in outdoor shelters.

GPS—Global Positioning Satellite systems are used to track individuals or vehicles. See page 75 for additional information.

Hallucinations—Sensations (visions, smells, sounds, tastes, or physical feelings) experienced entirely by, and within the mind of, the patient. Hallucinations have no visible clues to those of us on the outside.

Illusions—Misinterpretations of people, places or things.

Law Enforcement Personnel—Some communities are served by police departments, while others are served by sheriff's departments or sheriff's offices. To simplify this diversity, "law enforcement personnel," in this workbook, will refer to any and all police or sheriff's department/office personnel or agencies with law enforcement missions.

---

1. National Institute for Elopement Prevention and Resolution, www.elopement.org.

Mantrackers—Individuals who are specially trained and experienced in search techniques, discovering, evaluating and following clues leading to the whereabouts of missing or evasive people. They often are members of Search & Rescue units that have simply taken on a specialty, just as other members may have become dog handlers, etc.

MMSE—The Mini-Mental State Examination is the most commonly used test for complaints of memory problems or when a diagnosis of dementia is being considered. The maximum score is 30. A score below 24 indicates probable cognitive impairment; a score below 17 indicates definite cognitive impairment.

Pica—a pattern of eating inappropriate non-nutritive substances (such as dirt or paper).

PIO—The Public (or Press) Information Officer is the member of the law enforcement team who is responsible for providing information to the press, media coordination and news releases, and may act as a spokesman for the law enforcement department.

Scoot—a means of propelling oneself in a wheelchair using one's feet.

Sundowning or Sundown Syndrome—Agitation, irritability, increased confusion or difficulties (including understanding and communication) that typically occur later in the day or at night. (Refer also to page 6.)

Wandering—The term "wandering" is a generic term that refers to a number of activities and behaviors—from seemingly aimless meandering, to a purposeful stroll, to pacing, to a dedicated attempt to go somewhere. In essence we all wander, every day. However, the most serious type of wandering with regard to Alzheimer's disease or dementia is "elopement"—attempting to leave home, unable or unwilling to return.

Often when a person with Alzheimer's is said to be "wandering," what is meant is that he is lost and not able to return home—he has "eloped." "Elopement" is a life-threatening behavior for someone with dementia. (Refer also to the definition for "elopement.")

ACRONYMS AND ABBREVIATIONS

AD—Alzheimer's Disease

ADL—Activity of Daily Living

ALF—Assisted Living Facility

BOLO—"Be On the Lookout"

CJD—Creutzfeld-Jacob Disease

DAT—Dementia of the Alzheimer's Type

DNR—Do Not Resuscitate

ENR—Emergency Medical Responder

FLIR—Forward Looking Infrared

FTD—Frontal Lobe (Frontotemporal) Dementia

GPS—Global Positioning Satellite

LKP—Last Known Position (similar to PLS)

LO—Loved one or the subject person with AD

MMSE—Mini-Mental State Examination

NCIC—National Crime Information Center

PIO—Public/Press Information Officer

PLS—Point (or Place) Last Seen

SAR—Search and Rescue

NOTES

Part 13

Sources of Wander-Alerting Products

Sources of Wander-Alerting Products

Door Alarms and Motion Detectors

The Alzheimer's Store— www.alzstore.com or call (800) 752-3238

Perimeter and Distance Monitors

Care Electronics—www.careelectronics.com or call (888) 444-8284

Locator Systems Corporation—www.locatorsystemscorp.com or call (866) 863-5155

Project Lifesaver—www.projectlifesaver.org or call (757) 546-5502

Emergency Caller Products—www.emergencycaller.com or call (800) 227-2474

Automatic Dialers

Emergency Caller Products—www.emergencycaller.com or call (800) 227-2474

HomeFree—www.homefreesys.com or call (800) 606-0661

Locator Systems Corporation—www.locatorsystemscorp.com or call (866) 863-5155

Selective Alarms and Door Locking Devices

HomeFree—www.homefreesys.com or call (800) 606-0661

R.F. Technologies—www.codealert.com or call (800) 669-9946

Secure Care Products—www.securecare.com or call (800) 451-7917

Senior Technologies—www.seniortechnologies.com or call (800) 824-7140

SMART Caregiver Corporation—www.antiwandering.com or call (800) 650-3637

Xmark Systems—www.xmarksystems.com or call (866) 559-6275

Trackable Wander-Alert Systems

Care Electronics—www.careelectronics.com or call (888) 444-8284

Locator Systems Corporation—www.locatorsystemscorp.com or call (866) 863-5155

Project Lifesaver—www.projectlifesaver.org or call (757) 546-5502

Tracker Radio (Trackable system only—no alarm capabilities)—www.trackerradio.com or call (800) 900-2113

GPS Wander Alerting Devices

Wherify—www.wherifywireless.com or call (877) 943-7439

Refer to the In Search of the Alzheimer's
Wanderer website (www.alzwanderer.com)
for additional products and information.

Part 14

Resources and
Suggested Reading

Resources and Suggested Reading

Alzheimer's Association—The Alzheimer's Association is a national organization dedicated to finding preventions, treatments and a cure for Alzheimer's. Their mission is to eliminate the disease through the advancement of research and to enhance care and support for individuals, their families and caregivers. For more information on the Alzheimer's Association go to www.alz.org or call (800) 272-3900. You can also call this number to be connected to your local Alzheimer's Association chapter.

The Alzheimer's Foundation of America (AFA)—The Alzheimer's Foundation of America is a national organization whose mission is "to provide optimal care and services to individuals confronting dementia, and to their caregivers and families—through member organizations dedicated to improving quality of life." For more information about AFA go to www.alzfdn.org or call them at (866) 232-8484.

(The) Alzheimer's Store—The Alzheimer's Store provides products for people with Alzheimer's disease and those caring for them (including motion detectors, door alarms and other products to prevent or detect wandering). To contact The Alzheimer's Store or to request a free catalog go to www.alzstore.com or call (800) 752-3238.

The Complete Guide to Alzheimer's-Proofing Your Home, Mark L. Warner, Purdue University Press (2nd edition, 2000). This book offers many ideas and suggestions on how to create a safer home for people with Alzheimer's disease and related dementia disorders (available at The Alzheimer's Store www.alzstore.com or call (800) 752-3238).

Dementia and Wandering Behavior, Nina M. Silverstein, Gerald Flaherty, Terri Salmons Tobin, Springer Publishing Co., 2002. (available at The Alzheimer's Store www.alzstore.com or call (800) 752-3238).

Gone ... Without a Trace, Marianne Dickerman Caldwell (Elder Books, 1995) (available at The Alzheimer's Store, www.alzstore.com or call (800) 752-3238).

Studies on Wandering

To read full reports on studies involving wandering go to the following web sites:

Antecedents, descriptions and consequences of wandering in cognitively-impaired adults and the Safe Return Program, Meredeth A. Rowe, RN, PhD, Judith C. Glover, RN, MS—http://con.ufl.edu/dementia/ajadop166nd01.pdf

A look at deaths occurring in persons with dementia lost in the community, Meredeth A. Rowe, RN, PhD, Vikki Bennett, BSN—http://con.ufl.edu/dementia/ajadop186ndred01.pdf

"Lost Alzheimer's Subjects—Profiles and Statistics," R. J. Koester, D. E. Stooksbury, *Response* 11:4:20–26, 1992—http://www.dbs-sar.com/SAR_Research/response.pdf

"Behavioral Profile of Possible Alzheimer's Disease Subjects in Search and Rescue Incidents in Virginia," R. J. Koester, D. E. Stooksbury, *Wilderness and Environmental Medicine* 6:34–43, 1995—http://www.dbs-sar.com/SAR_Research/WEM_article.htm

Urban Search for an Alzheimer's Patient, Neil Brewer, Kent-Harrison Search & Rescue—http://www.sarinfo.bc.ca/alzheimerSOP.htm

For more information on finding lost persons with Alzheimer's disease, updates on found Alzheimer's wanderers, and added information to this book, please go to www.alzwanderer.com.

Contributors to This Book

Kimberly R. Kelly Falconer—Founder and executive director of Project Far From Home, a national not-for-profit educational program designed to teach law enforcement and search and rescue teams about missing at-risk Alzheimer's and dementia subjects. She is also a certified technical rescue specialist, reserve sergeant and SAR volunteer with the San Diego County Sheriff's Department. Sarlady@yahoo.com

Robert Koester—One of the nation's leading authorities on finding people with Alzheimer's disease who have wandered away from home or become lost. He is president of dbS Productions, which specializes in instructing and assisting Search and Rescue personnel find people with Alzheimer's disease. Robert@dbS-sar.com

Meredeth A. Rowe, RN, PhD—An expert on wandering with regard to people with Alzheimer's disease. She is the author of numerous studies on wandering and noted for her knowledge involving characteristics and data pertaining to found wanderers. Mrowe@ufl.edu

Gene Saunders—Chief Executive Officer for Project Lifesaver, an organization responsible for the safe return of more than 1200 wandering Alzheimer's patients. Project Lifesaver has a 100% recovery rate, with all persons found alive and returned home safely (most within 30 minutes). Gsaunders@projectlifesaver.org

Dotty St. Amand—Executive Director of The Alvin A. Dubin Alzheimer's Resource Center, a United Way organization which provides assistance and support to Alzheimer's persons and their caregivers in Lee County, Florida. DottySt@msn.com

John Thames—Family & Community Services Director for the Georgia Chapter of the Alzheimer's Association. His responsibilities include assisting and responding to emergencies involving the state's Safe Return Program. John.Thames@alz.org

Additional Notes

Additional Notes

Additional Notes

Additional Notes

Additional Notes

Additional Notes

MARK L. WARNER

the complete guide to

ALZHEIMER'S

Proofing Your Home

"The definitive guide for families with Alzheimer's and those professionals who counsel them."
—Beth McLeod, Author,
Caregiving: The Spiritual Journey of Love, Loss, and Renewal

"A superlative resource for home caregivers."
—*Booklist*

"Every family facing Alzheimer's and related dementia should also find a means to change..."
—Beverly Murphy, Author,
He Used to Be Somebody: A Journey into Alzheimer's Disease through the Eyes of a Caregiver

New paperback edition!
Revised and updated.

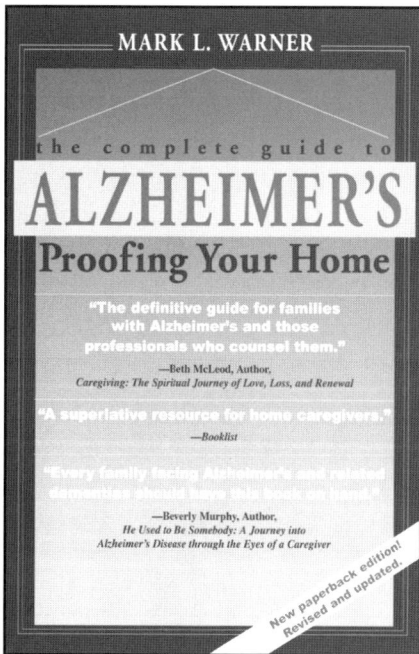

ISBN 1-55753-202-8

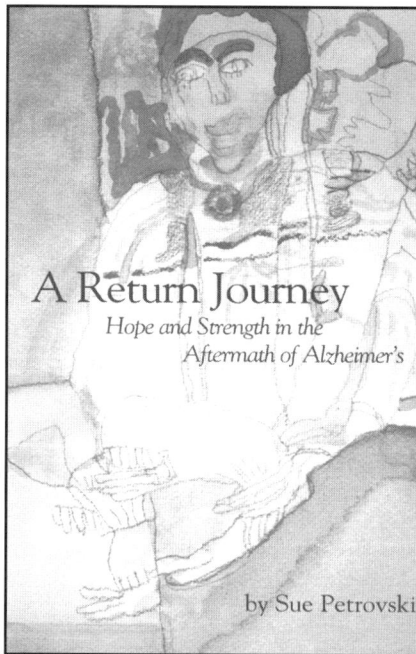

A Return Journey

Hope and Strength in the
Aftermath of Alzheimer's

by Sue Petrovski

ISBN 1-55753-302-4

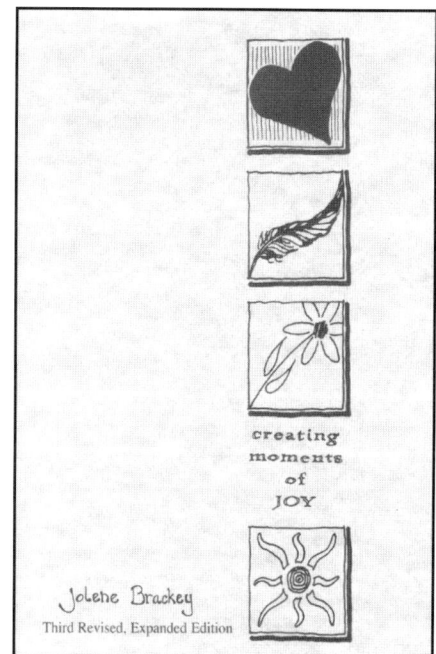

---

creating
moments
of
JOY

Jolene Brackey
Third Revised, Expanded Edition

ISBN 1-55753-366-0

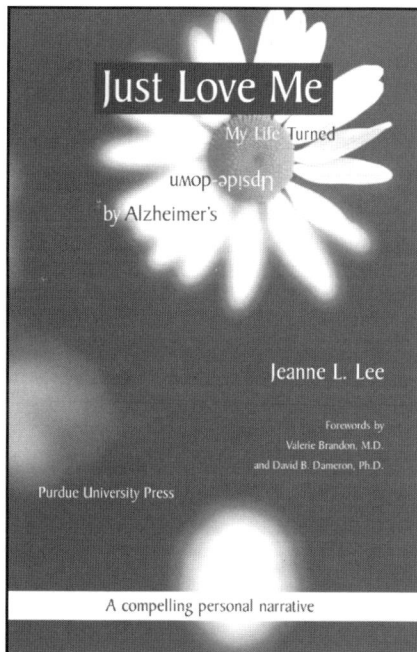

Just Love Me

My Life Turned
Upside-down
by Alzheimer's

Jeanne L. Lee

Forewords by
Valerie Brandon, M.D.
and David B. Dameron, Ph.D.

Purdue University Press

A compelling personal narrative

ISBN 1-55753-298-2

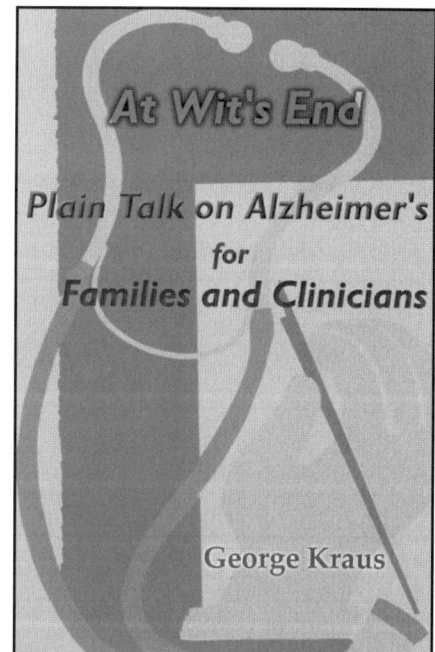

At Wit's End

Plain Talk on Alzheimer's
for
Families and Clinicians

George Kraus

ISBN 1-55753-401-2

PURDUE UNIVERSITY PRESS

1-800-247-6553

www.thepress.purdue.edu